Advance praise for *Between*

"A thoughtful, clear, conversational guide to the intricacies of medical science, studies and statistics. Any journalist who reports on the medical literature should keep a copy close by." — Maryn McKenna, MSJ, author of *SUPERBUG: The Fatal Menace of MRSA* and *BEATING BACK THE DEVIL: On the Front Lines with the Disease Detectives of the Epidemic Intelligence Service*

"Understanding how to read clinical studies critically is given short shrift in most medical and journalism schools, despite how important that skill is to reporters who write about science and doctors who help patients make decisions. Luckily, there are people like Marya Zilberberg to make up for that. Her blog Healthcare, etc. is a must read for medical and journalism students, and this book should be, too." — Ivan Oransky, MD, Executive Editor, Reuters Health; Adjunct Associate Professor of Journalism, New York University; Co-Founder of the science watchdog blog "Retraction Watch"

"*Between the Lines* should be required reading for *all* medical communications professionals and healthcare journalists. I'd even go further and say that understanding the material covered in BTL should be required for anyone involved in peer-review for medical journals or healthcare journalism." — Janice McCallum, Managing Director, Health Content Advisors

"Zilberberg walks the reader briskly through the assumptions, trade-offs and meanings of different types of health-related evidence. Whether you are patient with no statistical background who has just realized that you need to know this stuff or a savvy advocate with a couple biostats courses in your background, *Between the Lines* will, with clarity and humor, orient you to the basics of what you need to look out for when trying to make sense of the results of health research." — Jessie Gruman, PhD, President, Center for Advancing Health

"Dr. Zilberberg's book, *Between the Lines*, is provocative in challenging the meaning and application of published clinical evidence. She brings her extensive knowledge, and perspective encouraging readers to probe and question. ... *Between the Lines* provides a framework for a systematic approach to the medical literature and its application to practice, without which it is too easy to make the evidence fit our beliefs or cast it aside if it does not. That rational framework is as useful and important to me as a physician in industry as it would have been for me in the office or at my patients' hospital bedside. Dr. Zilberberg is also quite clear that the patient needs to be at the center of every decision and an active participant in the patient-physician partnership." — Roslyn Schneider, MD, MSc, FACP, FCCP, Senior Director, Medical Affairs, Pfizer Inc.

[*Dr. Schneider's opinion expressed here is her own and does not necessarily reflect that of Pfizer Inc.*]

Between the Lines

Between the Lines

Finding the Truth in Medical Literature

Marya Zilberberg, MD, MPH

E

EviMed Research Press
GOSHEN • MASSACHUSETTS

ISBN 978-0-9854562-0-7

Edited by Judith Cardanha
Cover design by Alex Hiam and Maggie Dana
Interior design and typesetting by Pageworks Press
Cover photo by Melanie Dana
Published by Evi*Med* Research Press, an imprint of Evi*Med*
Research Group, LLC, P.O. Box 303, Goshen, MA 01032
http://evimedgroup.com

for Melanie

Acknowledgments

There are many people to whom I owe a debt of gratitude. My family inspires me to learn every day and encourages me to share my ideas with the world. My mentors Scott Epstein and Leonard Sicilian taught me that the best clinicians make use of both the art and the science of medicine. My colleague and friend Andrew Shorr of the Washington Hospital Center has served as a sounding board for many of the ideas presented in this book; our discussions always serve to sharpen my understanding of methods and conclusions. My former boss and perennial mentor Catherine Tak Piech is in no small way responsible for this volume: She has always supported and cheered my pursuit of knowledge. My colleague Sandy Sulsky has participated in innumerable hours of discussion about the philosophical underpinnings of science.

Several professors at the University of Massachusetts School of Public Health and Health Sciences deserve mention: Susan Sturgeon welcomed and encouraged me to enter the Masters in Public Health program at the University of Massachusetts. Phil Nasca, who is currently the Dean of the University at Albany's School of Public Health, is the person who demystified all of the threats to validity that I address in this book. Carol Bigelow and Elizabeth Bertone-Johnson have spent time discussing with me the complexities of effect modification; and Melissa Troester, now back at her alma mater, the University of North Carolina at Chapel Hill, helped me clarify all of the ways to adjust for confounding. I am especially grateful to Dan Gerber, the Associate Dean for Academic Affairs at the University of Massachusetts School of Public Health and Health Sciences, for encouraging me to teach in the graduate program and to share my ideas with the future public health professionals.

I owe a special debt of gratitude to the readers of my blog, *Healthcare, etc.,* and to my students, who over the years have pushed me to the limits of my knowledge and thinking. Without them there would be very little content between the covers of this book.

Contents

Introduction

Thick March snow is piling up outside my office window while I am hard at work putting finishing touches on this manuscript. I take a break to click over to the table of contents in today's issue of the *New England Journal of Medicine*, and almost immediately I am captured by the intriguing title of a Perspectives piece: "What's the Alternative? The Worldwide Web of Integrative Medicine."[1] I read it, and I am amazed at how pertinent it is to the overarching goal of this volume.

In her piece, Srivastava, who is an oncologist from Australia, weaves a sorry tale of a young mother who, through a series of events, came to be screened by an unethical quack for circulating tumor cells in her blood. The test turned up positive; she was told that

---

[1]Srivastava, R. What's the Alternative? The Worldwide Web of Integrative Medicine. *New England Journal of Medicine* 2012; 366:783–785

she had advanced lung cancer and was given intra-
venous vitamin C at a cost of $6,000. Eventually she
ended up in the article author's office, where no evidence of cancer could be found. The author seems to
suggest that policy measures to regulate what she refers
to as "alternative medicine" would be the solution to
this conundrum. But is that really so? Has regulation of
the medical field assured integrity and patient safety?
Let's examine the evidence.

Medicine is one of the most heavily regulated fields
in the United States. Yet in 1999 the Institute of Medicine's report *To Err Is Human* uncovered nearly
100,000 deaths caused by errors in U.S. hospitals an-
nually. A few years later, we heard that infections contracted in hospitals cause nearly as many deaths. At the
same time the volume of discussion about the demand
for overdiagnosis and overtreatment and their perils
has been getting higher. While regulation can mitigate
some of these harms, it cannot extinguish them completely. The real answer lies in education and empowerment.

The fury of the recent controversies surrounding
screening for such diseases as breast and prostate cancers underscores the feelings of betrayal that the public
feels when uncertainty is injected into dearly held
truths. It reflects the failure of many people to understand, at least in some minimal way, the philosophical
underpinnings and the method of science. Every scientific advance brings with it many more questions than

answers; and as these questions are answered, new questions and new understandings arise. Science is fluid and uncertain and beautiful that way, and it should make all of us constantly question all of our assumptions.

But science can also seem intimidating and daunting and inaccessible. And as news outlets continue to pump out breathless reports of medical breakthroughs that make it look as if immortality were just around the corner, both lay people and those trained in the clinical sciences are put off by the escalating complexity of medical literature and leave truth finding to others. Such abdication is fraught with consequences, since those who are charged with interpretation and decision making are, on the one hand, not always equipped to do it and, on the other, view the task through the prisms of their own values and experiences. And, yes, clinical science is sufficiently imprecise to lend itself to such varied conclusions. How often have you heard the warning "Buyer beware"?

I have been sailing the seas of evidence-based medicine for nearly two decades, teaching methods of evaluation, serving as a peer reviewer and an editorial board member for several medical journals, and most recently blogging. All these years and activities have led me to believe that we can do much better: We can do better research, we can be better peer reviewers and editors, and we can be better readers and interpreters of the data. In this era of information overload, the incredibly shrinking medical appointment, and the emergence of the e-patient movement, being well-versed in the methods is no longer optional.

This book is here to help. It is intended to give you some basic tools with which to examine medical literature critically and systematically, to develop your own interpretation toolbox instead of relying solely on that of others. This is a toolbox that you can open every time you are faced with making a medical decision, so that, unlike the young mother in the *New England Journal* article, you can guard against charlatans of all stripes.

Who should read this book? Who shouldn't? The current model of disseminating medical information relies on a layer of translators—journalists and clinicians. But I believe that every educated person must at the very least understand how these interpreters of medical knowledge examine, or *should* examine, it to arrive at the conclusions that ultimately make their way to the public. At the same time, both journalists and clinicians may benefit from this refresher. Based on news releases that I have seen describing studies, this volume is a must-read for the public relations professionals who develop those releases. Medical librarians may find this book particularly helpful: Being at the forefront of evidence dissemination, they can lead the charge of separating credible science from rubbish. Similarly, biopharmaceutical professionals within Medical Affairs groups, specifically those in the Medical

Science Liaison roles, have found the ideas in this book helpful when I have presented them in workshops and seminars. Finally, one of my professional goals is to help improve the surprisingly variable quality of peer review in clinical literature. So, I particularly encourage new peer reviewers for clinical journals to read on.

A few words on the format of the book: I have purposely kept my tone conversational and references to a minimum, since most of the ideas that will be discussed are well accepted. When citations are unavoidable, I have made them fairly unobtrusive by putting them in the footnotes. I have also tried to keep computations low-key, focusing instead on conveying broad concepts. Furthermore, I have tried not to get into minutia or to explain everything to its limit, as fuller explanations, when needed, are easily accessed in more comprehensive texts. For these reasons, I am not expecting that this work will replace a course on how research is carried out and evaluated. But I do hope to make the reader aware of what a critical review of a paper looks like.

The book consists of two parts. Part One serves to set the stage for how we should think about science, particularly the science that informs the practice of clinical medicine. It is a compilation of short essays on some general concepts that interfere with the process of posing and giving rational answers to questions in medicine. Here we will touch on how shortcuts in thinking and cognitive biases make us prone to misinterpreting data. We will also make a brief detour into some philosophical issues that define scientific method, particularly as applied to clinical research. And most important, we will take a close look at *uncertainty* as the only certain feature of science and learn how to get comfortable with it.

Part Two is concerned with the fundamentals of evaluation, the tools that should be in the toolbox of everyone who wants to know what to make of a finding. We will examine ways to evaluate the components of a study: question, design, analyses, results, reporting, and conclusions.

For this journey, we will look at different studies to examine many different types of study designs. I have, however, chosen the landmark Women's Health Initiative study that reported on the risks and benefits of menopausal hormone replacement therapy as a recurring guide throughout this discussion.[2] This study is available on the JAMA web site for free (see footnote for the link), and you can access it for yourself, should you want to navigate along with me. I will refer to it as "WHI-HRT" when discussing certain general points of

---

[2]Writing group for the Women's Health Initiative Investigators. Risks and Benefits -of Estrogen Plus Progestin in Healthy Postmenopausal Women: Principal Results from the Women's Health Initiative Randomized Controlled Trial. *JAMA* 2002; 288:321–333 Available at http://jama.ama-assn.org/content/288/3/321.full.pdf+html

medical literature, as well as in some specific instances when dealing with evidence.

Some of the things I say may seem contradictory at first: I may in one sentence extol the virtues of a randomized controlled trial and in the next knock it down. I may then proceed to tell you why observational studies lack certain elements of validity and shortly thereafter hold them up as an example of good research. There is a simple reason for this apparent contradiction: No study is perfect, all designs have strengths and weaknesses, and there is just no shortcut to knowing how to recognize them.

And that is the whole point of this book. I hope that reading and using it prevents you from falling prey to any kind of predatory quackery, be it "alternative medicine" or overly zealous disease mongering by the medical establishment. If there is only one thing you take away from this volume, it should be this: Every decision you make comes with risks and benefits. Do not let anyone with a vested interest pull wool over your eyes and blind you to these risks.

And one last thing: When I was growing up, I was taught that it was disrespectful to write in books. Well, I encourage you to write, underline, highlight, dog-ear, and leave sticky notes in this book (provided it belongs to you). I cannot imagine a more eloquent show of respect.

PART ONE

Context

MUCH OF OUR CURRENT DISCOURSE does not do justice to the complexity of ideas we face within medicine every day. Neither the press nor academic reductionism can possibly capture this complexity fairly. We are faced with rampant uncertainties, which make science so exciting.

This part of the book consists of essays that help us put in perspective science in general and clinical science in particular. These essays will likely frustrate you by raising questions that may not have convenient answers. To me, this is the essence and the beauty of science.

CHAPTER 1

The Importance of Denominators

Let's face it: Denominators keep numbers and the people reporting them honest. Imagine if I said that there were 3,352 cases of a never-before-seen strain of flu in the United States. To be sure, 3,352 cases is a large enough number to send us rushing to buy a respirator mask. But what if I put it slightly differently and said that out of the population of roughly 300,000,000 individuals, 3,352 have contracted this strain of flu? I think this makes things a little different, since it means that the risk of contracting the flu to date is about 1 in 100,000, a fairly low number as risks go.

Now, I am going to give you another number: 86. This represents the number of the novel H1N1 flu-related deaths in Mexico reported on April 25, 2009, by the health minister of Mexico. At that time this flu had been thought to have sickened 1,400 people. This puts the risk of death from the flu at roughly 6%, a very high risk indeed! Well, that was then.

After the health authorities had gone back and done some testing, as of May 12, 2009, Mexico had confirmed 2,059 flu cases with 56 fatalities, equating to a 2.7% risk of dying from the disease—still a high number, but lower than what had been thought before.

In the United States, as of May 12, 2009, there were 3 fatalities among 3,352 reported flu cases, yielding the risk of death from H1N1 in this country at that time at about 1 in 1,000. But, of course, the denominator of 3,352 persons represented only those who had sought medical attention and been tested; so it was almost certainly an underestimate of the true burden of this strain of flu and thus also an overestimate of its attendant mortality. Now, apply this to the situation in Mexico, and it's likely that the risk of death from H1N1 was also lower than what had been observed, precisely due to the underestimation of the denominator.

So how could we have gotten a true estimate of the numbers of people afflicted with the H1N1 influenza? Well, we could have screened absolutely everyone (or, more likely, a large and representative group of individuals). And then what? Would we treat them all with antiviral medications? Would we observe them? Since the Centers for Disease Control and Prevention had recommended testing only severe cases and treating only people at a high risk for complications, universal testing did not seem like a practical approach. Furthermore, as you will see in Chapters 3 and 4, testing people without any symptoms is fraught with false positive results followed by overtreatment. So, the bottom line is that we were not likely during the H1N1 pandemic to get at the correct denominator for the risk of dying from exposure to this virus and that any number that we did get was likely an overestimate of the true risk.

A more recent example of how important denominators are comes from a paper published in *Science*.[3] Here the authors performed a pooled analysis of studies to determine the prevalence of exposure to avian influenza, or the H5N1 virus. Their data indicated that exposure rates to this virus are much higher than previously thought, thus substantially increasing the denominator of people at risk for death from this bug. And clearly, when the denominator (people at risk for the outcome) goes up and the numerator (the outcome, death) remains the same, the inevitable conclusion is that the deadly nature of the virus may have been overstated.

What are the lessons here? First, don't let anyone get away with only giving you the numerator, as that is not

[3]Wang, T. T., Parides, M. K., & Palese, P. Seroevidence for H5N1 Influenza Infections in Humans: Meta-Analysis. *Science*, published online February 23, 2012.

even half the story. Second, even when the denominator appears known, be skeptical: Does it really represent the entire pool of cases that are at risk for the event that the numerator describes? Clearly, the denominator is the key to being an educated consumer of health information.

CHAPTER 2

When Do Diagnostic Tests Save Lives?

The title question is well worth asking, particularly as the argument about the merits of mammography screening continues. The United States Preventive Services Task Force (USPSTF) really stirred up a hornet's nest with their recent recommendations.[4] But the question remains: Do screening or diagnostic tests that are more sensitive save lives?

A terrific paper examining this issue was published in the *Archives of Internal Medicine* in May 2011. The subject of the study was pulmonary embolism (PE), or

---

[4]US Preventive Services Task Force. Screening for breast cancer: US Preventive Services Task Force recommendation statement. *Annals of Internal Medicine* 2009; 151:716–726

a clot that can migrate to someone's lungs and cause potentially life-threatening complications.[5] The traditional way of detecting this condition prior to the late 1990s was to run a special type of a scan, which was neither particularly sensitive nor specific. Thus, its interpretation relied largely on what the clinician thought was the patient's pre-test probability of a PE. This reliance on the clinical situation was somewhat relaxed with the introduction in 1998 of CT angiography for detecting this condition. And while this technology raised the sensitivity, thus allowing the detection of more PEs, it also reduced the specificity thus promoting overdiagnosis by increasing the risk of identifying PEs that are not of any clinical consequence.

The concern over this overly sensitive diagnostic test as a path to overdiagnosis of clinically insignificant disease led investigators at Dartmouth to conduct the PE study I mentioned earlier. The thesis they posed was simple: If the CT angiography is helping to detect more clinically significant PEs, then PE-related mortality should have decreased over time, just as the technology is detecting more PEs. Their findings were sobering, albeit not unexpected. But before I spell out for you what those findings were, you need to understand measures of mortality a little better.

---

[5]Weiner, R. S., Schwartz, L. M., & Woloshin, S. Time Trends in Pulmonary Embolism in the United States: Evidence of Overdiagnosis. *Archives of Internal Medicine* 2011; 171:831–837

We have heard that mortality from many diseases has decreased over the past few decades. But is this true? To answer that question, we have to ask what is meant by *mortality*. Even people well versed in epidemiology and biostatistics occasionally blur the lines between mortality and case fatality, but to our question the distinction is critical. *Case fatality* is defined as the proportion of patients with the disease who die, whereas *mortality*, a population-based measure, is defined as the proportion of all the at-risk people who die from the disease. The difference lies in our old friend the denominator, which will always keep us honest.

Let's go through a simple example to illustrate this: Pretend that 30 years ago the total number of cases of disease D diagnosed using the stone-age test T was 100 in a population of 10,000 people. Of these cases, 90 died, giving us the *case fatality* of 90/100, or 90%, and *mortality* of 9 per 1,000 population (Figure 1a). Now, there is a new test for D, a super-Doppler-MRI-PET-cyberscan called über-T, a test that is much more sensitive than the old test T. With über-T, 1,000 cases of D are detected in the population of 10,000 people. Of those 1,000, 90 have died (Figure 1b). The case fatality now has decreased dramatically from 90% to 9% (90/1,000), and we can pat ourselves on the back for a job well done, right? Not so fast: The population mortality from disease D has remained a steady 9 per 1,000.

Figure 1 **Mortality versus Case Fatality**

Figure 1a

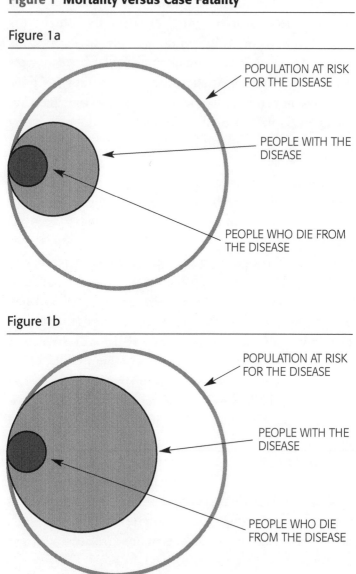

POPULATION AT RISK
FOR THE DISEASE

PEOPLE WITH THE
DISEASE

PEOPLE WHO DIE FROM
THE DISEASE

Figure 1b

POPULATION AT RISK
FOR THE DISEASE

PEOPLE WITH THE
DISEASE

PEOPLE WHO DIE
FROM THE DISEASE

What does this mean? Is the über-T, which costs two orders of magnitude more than its predecessor, worthless? Well, decide for yourselves. What it means to me is that detecting additional cases by the über-T amounts to overdiagnosis, which increases the denominator for the case-fatality calculation, but has had no impact on the numerator. Therefore, the über-T has not in fact improved the only mortality that matters: population mortality.

Going back to the Dartmouth PE study, the investigators indeed discovered that more PEs were diagnosed following the introduction of CT angiography. It is interesting that they also detected a small drop in mortality related to PE, from 12.3 to 11.9 per 100,000 population. But looking back at what had been happening to PE mortality in an earlier time period, they realized that this drop was much smaller in magnitude than the drop they had noted in the five years prior to the introduction of CT, which had gone from 13.4 to 12.3 per 100,000. This meant that whatever drop in mortality that occurred after the introduction of CT angiography paled in comparison to the drop that had occurred before, making a strong case for overdiagnosis as a result of using this new technology.

So, next time you hear how well a new test is doing in disease management, ask this simple question: Has it really altered the important outcomes, or is this all smoke and mirrors, a mirage created by our failure to examine critical questions critically? This may be an uncomfortable epiphany for some. But think about the 900 excess cases of the pseudo-disease diagnosed in our earlier example: How many people could have been spared a disease label and overtreatment, how many complications of follow-up procedures could have been avoided, and, yes, how much money could have been spent on something other than healthcare? And asking these questions may help us to identify true technological advances that actually improve our lives.

CHAPTER 3

Beware of What Seems Too Good to Be True

I recently came across an announcement that a company in California has come up with a breathalyzer-type device that can diagnose lung cancer with 83% accuracy.[6] This, the company claims, is a big improvement over currently existing diagnostics, which "result in too many false positives, meaning unnecessary biopsies and radiation imaging." And if this weren't enough, the company is purportedly testing an even more accurate version of the device, which will have a 90% diagnostic accuracy for lung cancer. Wow, forgive

---

[6]Jones, O. A Breathalyzer for Cancer. *Big Think* [blog]. Accessed February 16, 2012. Available at http://bigthink.com/ideas/42492

me if I am not getting, well, breathless about this. Neither should you, and here is why. There is no doubt that lung cancer is a devastating disease, and science has not done a great job reducing its burden or the associated mortality. However, there are several issues with what the California company is implying, and some of the assumptions are unclear. First, what does *accuracy* mean? In the world of epidemiology, it refers to how well the test identifies true positives and true negatives. If that is in fact what the story means, then 83% may not be bad (we'll regroup on that point later in this chapter).

Second, what is the gold standard against which the test is being measured? In other words, what is it that has the 100% accuracy in lung cancer detection? Is it a chest X-ray? a CT scan? a biopsy? The Surveillance, Epidemiology, and End Results (SEER) database maintained by the National Cancer Institute, one of the most rigorous sources of cancer statistics in the United States, classifies tissue diagnosis as the highest evidence of cancer. However, in some cases a clinical diagnosis is acceptable. The inference of cancer when no tissue is examined is possible when weighing patient risk factors and the behavior of the tumor. So, you see where I am going here? The gold standard is tissue or tumor behavior in a specific patient. Is that what this technology is being measured against? If not, if it is in fact being measured against a less accurate diagnostic, these inaccuracies get magnified to the point of "garbage in, garbage out."

But these issues are but a prelude to what is the real problem with a technology like the one described: the predictive value of a positive test. The announcement even alluded to this, pointing the finger at other current-day technologies and their rates of false positivity and away from itself. Yet, in fact, this is the crux of the matter for all diagnostics. Let me show you what I mean: According to the National Cancer Institute, the annual incidence of lung cancer in the United States is on the order of 60 cases per 100,000 population. Now, let us give this test a huge break and say that it yields (consistently) 99% *sensitivity* (identifies patients with cancer when cancer is really present) and 99% *specificity* (identifies patients without cancer when they really do not have cancer). To be sure, such sensitivity and specificity would be the envy of all. Table 1 shows what this will look like numerically if we test 100,000 people.

TABLE 1 Incidence 60 per 100,000, test sensitivity 99%, test specificity 99%

	Cancer present	Cancer absent	Total
Test +	59 (true positive)	999 (false positive)	1,058 (positive)
Test −	1 (false negative)	98,941 (true negative)	98,942 (negative)
Total	60 (have cancer)	99,940 (don't have cancer)	100,000 (screened)

If we add up all the "wrong" test results, the false negative (disease present, but test negative, $n = 1$) and the false positives (disease absent, but test positive, $n = 999$), we arrive at a 1% (1,058 ÷ 100,000) "inaccuracy" rate, or 99% accuracy. But what is hiding behind this 99% accuracy is the fact that of all those people with a positive test, only a handful, a paltry 6%, actually have cancer. And what does this mean for the other 94%? Additional testing, a lot of it invasive. And what does this testing mean for the healthcare system? You connect the dots.

Let's explore a slightly different scenario: Let us assume that there is a population of patients whose risk for developing lung cancer is 10 times higher than that of the population average. Let us say that their annual incidence is 600 cases per 100,000 population. Let us perform the same calculation again, assigning this same bionic accuracy to the test (Table 2).

The accuracy remains at 99%, but the value of the positive test rises to 37%. Still, 63% of all people test-

TABLE 2 Incidence 600 per 100,000, test sensitivity 99%, test specificity 99%

	Cancer present	Cancer absent	Total
Test +	594	994	1,588
Test –	6	98,406	98,412
Total	600	99,400	100,000

ing positive for cancer will go on to unnecessary testing. And imagine the numbers if millions of people were screened rather than just 100,000.

Let us do just one final calculation. Let us reflect the data back to the test in question, where the announcement claims that the accuracy of the next version of the technology will be 90%. Assuming a high-risk population (600 cases per 100,000 population), what does a positive result mean (Table 3)?

From this table, the accuracy is indeed 90%, concealing the very low value of a positive test of only 5%. This means that of the people testing positive for lung cancer with this technology, 95% will be false positives! For this high-risk group, what is most startling is that to arrive at the same mediocre 37% positive-test value that we saw previously, we would need a population where annual cancer incidence is a whopping 6,000 per 100,000, meaning that 6% of the population develops lung cancer every year!

What can we conclude? Screening for disease that is

TABLE 3 Incidence 600 per 100,000, test sensitivity 90%, test specificity 90%

	Cancer present	Cancer absent	Total
Test +	540	9,940	10,480
Test −	60	89,460	89,520
Total	600	99,400	100,000

not yet a clinical problem is fraught with many pitfalls, and manufacturers and the public need to be aware of these logic traps. There is an inexorable inverse tie between the pretest probability of a disease and the risk of a false positive result: The lower the former, the higher the latter. For this reason, as I have shown you here, even when the "accuracy" of a test is exquisitely (almost impossibly) high, it is the pre-test probability of, or the person's risk for, the disease that is the overwhelming driver of false positives. So, beware of tests that sound too good to be true—most of the time they are.

CHAPTER 4

Why Medical Testing Is Never a Simple Decision

Recently *Archives of Internal Medicine* published a case report.[7] It did this to highlight the theme "Less Is More" in medicine. The case involved a middle-aged woman presenting to the emergency room with vague symptoms of chest pain. Although from reading the paper it becomes clear that the pain is highly unlikely to represent heart disease, the doctors caring for the patient elected to do a non-invasive computed tomography (CT) angiography test, just to

---

[7]Becker, M. C., Galla, J. M., & Nissen, S. E. Left Main Trunk Coronary Artery Dissection as a Consequence of Inaccurate Coronary Computed Tomographic Angiography. *Archives of Internal Medicine* 2011; 171:698–701

"reassure" the patient, as the authors put it. Well, the test came back positive, the woman went for an invasive cardiac catheterization, where, though no disease was found, she suffered a very rare but devastating tear of one of the arteries in her heart. As you can imagine, she became very ill, required bypass surgery and, ultimately, an urgent heart transplant. It is startling to realize that she went from a healthy woman to a heart transplant patient in just a few weeks.

The case illustrates the pitfalls of getting a seemingly innocuous test for what appears to be a humanistic reason—patient reassurance. Yet, look at the tsunami of harm that followed this one decision. But what is done is done. The big question is, can cases like this be prevented? And if so, how? I will submit to you that Bayesian approaches to testing can and should reduce such complications. Here is how.

First, what is Bayesian thinking? *Bayesian thinking* in medicine refers to considering the probability of a condition existing when interpreting a subsequent event. One example is taking into account the probability of a disease being present when interpreting the result of a test for this disease. What does this mean? Well, let us take the much-embattled example of mammography and put some numbers to the probabilities. Assume that an otherwise healthy woman between 40 and 50 years of age has a 1% chance of developing breast cancer (that is, 1 out of every 100 such women, or 100 out of 10,000, undergoing screening). [Full disclosure: I am using 1% for ease of presentation; the actual risk in this age group is 1 in 70, or 1.4%.[8] But let's continue.] Now, suppose that a screening mammogram is able to pick up 80% of all cancers that are actually there (true positives), meaning that 20% go unnoticed by this technology. So, among the 100 women with actual breast cancer of the 10,000 women screened, 80 will be diagnosed as having cancer, while 20 will be missed.

Since no test in medicine is perfect, assume also that in a certain fraction of the screenings, mammography will merely imagine that a cancer is present, when in fact there is no cancer. Say that this happens about 10% of the time. So, going back to the 10,000 women being screened, of 9,900 who do NOT have cancer (remember that only 100 can have a true cancer), 10%, or 990 individuals, will still be diagnosed as having cancer. So, tallying up all of the positive mammograms, we are now faced with 1,070 women diagnosed with breast cancer. But, of course, of these women only 80 actually have the cancer. How can this be? We have arrived at the very important idea of the value of a positive test: This roughly tells us how sure we should be that a positive test actually means that the disease is present. It is a simple ratio of the real positives (true

[8]US Preventive Services Task Force. Screening for breast cancer: US Preventive Services Task Force recommendation statement. *Annals of Internal Medicine* 2009; 151:716–726

positives, in this case, the 80 women with true cancer) to all of the positives obtained with the test (in this case 1,070). This is called *positive predictive value* of a test; and in our mammography example for women between ages of 40 and 50, it turns out to be 7.5%. So, what this means is that out of 10 women told that their mammograms are abnormal, 9 will be told this based on a false positive result.

Now, let us look at the flip side of this equation, or the value of a negative test. Of the 8,930 negative mammograms, only 20 will be false negatives (remember that in this case mammography will only pick up 80 out of 100 true cancers). This means that the other 8,910 negative results are true negatives, making the value of a negative test, or negative predictive value, 8,910/8,930 = 99.8%, or just fantastic! So, if the test is negative, we can be pretty comfortable that there is no cancer. However, if the test is positive, while cancer is present in 80 women, 900 others will undergo unnecessary further testing. And for every subsequent test a similar calculus applies, since all tests are fallible.

Let's do one more maneuver. Say that now we have a population of 10,000 women who have a 10% chance of having breast cancer (as is the case with an older population). The sensitivity and specificity of mammography do not change, yet the positive and negative predictive values do. So, among these 10,000 women, 1,000 are expected to have cancer, of which 800 will be picked up on mammography. Among the 9,000 without cancer, a mammogram will "find" a cancer in 900. So, the total positive mammograms add up to 1,700, of which nearly 50% are true positives (800/1,700 = 47.1%). It is interesting that the negative predictive value does not change a whole lot (8,100/[8,100 + 200]) = 97.6%, or still quite acceptably high). So, while among younger women at a lower risk for breast cancer, a positive mammogram indicates the presence of disease in only 8% of the cases, for older women it is about 50% correct. And while this is better, as you can see, it is still far from perfect. This is why patients must understand these implications for their data and make informed choices based on what risks and what benefits matter most to them.

These two examples illustrate how exquisitely sensitive an interpretation of any test result is to the pre-test probability that a patient has the disease. Applying this to the woman in the case report in the *Archives*, some back-of-the-napkin calculations based on the numbers in the report itself suggest that while a negative CT angiogram would indeed have been reassuring, a positive one would only create confusion, as, in fact, it did.

Certainly, if we had a perfect test, or one that picked up disease 100% of the time when it was present and did not mislabel people without the disease as having it, we would not need to apply this type of Bayesian accounting. However, to the best of my knowledge, no such test exists in today's clinical practice, nor is it likely to exist in the future. Therefore, engaging in explicit calculations of what results can be expected in a particular patient from a particular test before ordering such a test can save a lot of headaches, and perhaps even lives. The new health information environments must have such risk algorithms built into all decision support systems. Bayesian probability is an idea whose time has surely come.

CHAPTER 5

Hierarchies and Causes

In the hierarchy of evidence, depending on where you look, it is either the meta-analysis or the *randomized controlled trial* (RCT) that is the gold standard. The latter is a great proof-of-concept tool, but it is necessarily limited in its external validity, or generalizability. The reason for this is that these trials—frequently done for regulatory approval to market a technology— enroll limited types of patients, exert extremely stringent controls on the total care of the patient (or else are criticized for not doing so), focus on short-term and surrogate outcomes (hence, the use of cholesterol lowering as a marker for cardiac mortality, for example) and usually do a fairly abysmal job of considering the sources of heterogeneity in the response rates and magnitudes. The interventions come to market and are typically used in a population that is either broader than or simply different from those enrolled in the RCT.

Many studies have documented this perennial problem with trial evidence, where real-world use of a therapy goes far beyond the available evidence. Certainly *meta-analyses*, which are a way to combine the data from multiple RCTs in a systematic way, when done well can give us greater confidence in the direction and the magnitude of the treatment effect; but they in no way overcome the generalizability issues of their component RCTs.

The next level in the evidence hierarchy is *observational data*, specifically cohort studies, first prospective, then retrospective. Cohort studies give us the opportunity to examine what happens in the real world without imposing the artificial conditions necessary in a clinical trial. Observational data can be great when describing epidemiology of a particular disease, the frequency of a given exposure, and the ways different characteristics can modify the relationship between the exposure and the outcome. One of the most attractive features of cohort studies is that the population can be observed over long periods of time—just look at the Nurses' Health Study, the Framingham Cohort, and others. But these types of studies also have important limitations, as we will see in Part Two of this book, and they are readily acknowledged as having a heightened susceptibility to bias (especially retrospective studies), the possibility of misclassifying important events, and, despite our best efforts to adjust for it, residual sources for confounding the data. I will come clean and admit my affection for observational data, even though it is considered a lower level of evidence than an RCT.

There are philosophical reasons to disagree that observational data are any less valuable than interventional data when it comes to the inference of causality. A paper by Rothman and Greenland that I like my students to read examines this in great detail and never fails to cause angst in the class.[9] And it is no wonder: One of the shocking headings in the paper is "Impossibility of Proof." You have to have nerves of steel not to get anxious contemplating something like this. The authors argue that this sentiment, which goes back to the eighteenth-century Scottish philosopher David Hume, who said that proof was not possible in an empirical science, applies to laboratory investigations and RCTs and not only to the science of epidemiology. Rothman and Greenland cleverly point out that many scientific discoveries, such as the theory of evolution, relied on observation alone. The ultimate point is that, no matter how close we think we get to the truth, all we can hope to construct is essentially a mental model of reality, and not reality itself. Indeed, we can get very close to it but

---

[9]Rothman, K. J., & Greenland, S. Causation and causal inference in epidemiology. *American Journal of Public Health* 2005; 95:S144–S150

never quite have it within our grasp. So, again, despite myriad caveats, observational data are no less valuable than results of experiments. The fact is that the two are complementary. It is like the fable of the blind men and the elephant: In isolation each perceives but a single part, while together the entire elephant emerges.

What follows cohort studies in the hierarchy of evidence are case-control studies, done usually when the outcome of interest is rare. Then come case reports and, finally, expert opinion. When evidence-based guidelines are developed, a comprehensive systematic literature review is undertaken, and the totality of evidence is examined and ranked. Based on these papers, a recommendation is made, and the strength of this recommendation is reported, taking into account the quality of the underlying evidence. This is an arduous and costly process, and it is commendable that it is undertaken. At the same time, given the limitations of the components of the guideline, the final product is only as good as its parts. I believe in the scientific method, yet I am simply not convinced that researchers have done such a great job generating trustworthy evidence in many instances. At the same time, I am not totally nihilistic about what we know; the truth lies somewhere between thinking that we understand everything perfectly and thinking that we know nothing. The heated debates in which scientists and clinicians engage are a testament exactly to how not straightforward our science is. I also understand that as a researcher I can afford a certain amount of analysis paralysis that is unacceptable at the bedside. However, I think we (and the press) do a disservice to patients, to ourselves, and to the science if we are not upfront about just how uncertain much of what we think we know is. Sherry Boschert, a science journalist and the author of the book *Plug-in Hybrids*,** recently summarized this view:[10]

"It would be nice if we could all agree that science is not static, but rather progresses and regresses. We learn, and then find out that some of what we thought we had learned was wrong, and set about using that information to seek the next level of truth. Repeat, *ad infinitum*. Personally, I'd love it if my doctors couched every bit of advice with, 'Here's what we think we know today.'

But I suspect that wouldn't sit well with many patients, who want certainty (as if there is such a thing). And it especially seems like a difficult proposition in our contentious society, where anti-science nay-sayers like to jump on contradictory findings to challenge the basic value of science overall."

---

[10]Boschert, S. Science Gets It Wrong and Right. *EGMN: Notes from the Road* blog, accessed October 21, 2010. Available at http://egmnblog.wordpress.com/2010/10/21/science-gets-it-wrong-and-right/

**Gabriola Island, BC, Canada: New Society Publishers, 2006.

CHAPTER 6

Assume a Spherical Cow

You know that joke about the farmer whose cows are not producing enough milk? A university panel gathers under the leadership of a theoretical physicist. They analyze each aspect of the problem thoroughly and carefully and, after much deliberation, produce a report, the first line of which is, "First, assume a spherical cow in a vacuum." This joke has become shorthand for some of the reductionist thinking in theoretical physics, but it can just as easily personify the field of statistics, on which we rely so heavily to inform our evidence-based practices.

Here is what I mean. Let us look at four common applications of statistical principles. First, *descriptive statistics*, usually represented by "Table 1" in a paper, are intended to help us understand the measures of central tendency, such as the mean and median values. I would argue that both measures are somewhat flawed in the real world. As we all learned, a mean is a bona fide measure of central tendency in a normal or Gaussian distribution. And furthermore, in such a distribution, 95% confidence intervals are bounded by 2.5× the standard deviation from the mean. Although this is very convenient, few things about human biology are actually distributed normally; many cluster to the left or to the right of the center, creating a tail on the opposite end. For these skewed distributions a median is the recommended measure to be used, bracketed by the boundaries of the 25% to 75% range of the values, or the interquartile range. But in a skewed distribution it is exactly the tail that is its most telling feature, as described so eloquently and personally by Stephen J. Gould in his "The Median Isn't the Message" essay.[11] This is especially true when more specific identification of characteristics causes the numbers to dwindle; for example, if instead of such general measures as blood pressure among all comers, you want to focus on morning blood pressures in such a specific group as African-American males with a history of diabetes and hypercholesterolemia who attend a smoking cessation program.

---

[11]Gould, S. J. The median isn't the message. Available at http://people.umass.edu/biep540w/pdf/Stephen%20Jay%20 Gould.pdf

Second, *analytic modeling* relies on the assumption of normality. To overcome this limitation, we transform certain non-normal distributions to their logarithm forms, for example, to normalize them in order to force them to play nicely. Once normalized, we perform the prestidigitation of a regression, reverse-transform the outcome to its anti-log, and, voila, you have an undisputable result! And even though statisticians tend to argue about such techniques, in the real world of research, where evidence cannot wait for perfection, we accept this legerdemain as the best we can do.

Third is *pooled analyses*, specifically meta-analyses. The intent of meta-analyses is to present the totality of evidence in a single convenient and easily comprehended value. One specific circumstance in which a meta-analysis is considered useful occurs when different studies are in conflict with one another, as, for example, when one study demonstrates that an intervention is effective, whereas another does not show such effectiveness. In my humble opinion, it is one thing to pool data when studies are just too small to detect a significant result. It is another thing, however, if the studies simply show opposite results. What if one study indicates a therapeutic advantage of treatment T over placebo P, but another study shows the exact opposite? Is it still valid to combine these studies to get at the "true" story? Or is it better to leave them separate and try to understand the potential differences in the study designs, populations, interventions, measurements, and outcomes? I am not saying that all meta-analyses mislead us, but I do think that in the wrong hands this technique can be dangerous, smoothing out differences that are potentially critical. This is one spherical cow that needs to be milked before it is bought.

Fourth is the one-on-one *patient-clinician encounter,* wherein the doctor needs to cram the multidimensional individual patient, with his/her ambiguous predispositions, into the spherical container of evidence. It is here that all of the other cows are magnified to obscene proportions to create a cumbersome, at times incomprehensible, and frequently useless pile of manure. It is one thing for a clinician to ignore evidence willfully; it is entirely another to be a conscientious objector to what is known but not applicable to the individual in the office.

But let's remember that manure holds life-giving properties. Extending the metaphor then, this pile of manure can and should be used to fertilize our field of knowledge by viewing each therapeutic encounter systematically as its own experiment. The middle way is the one between the cynicism of discarding and the gullibility of blindly accepting any and all evidence. That is where the art of medicine must come in, and the emerging payment systems must take it into account. Doctors need time, intellectual curiosity, and skills to conduct these individual-patient (also known as "n of 1") trials in their offices. This is the surest way to direct

"conscientious and judicious" application of the resulting oceans of population data in the service of our
public's health if new data insist on continuing to come
in tidal waves. And that should make the farmer happy,
even if his cows are spherical.

CHAPTER 7

Why Some Blockbuster Drugs Don't Work for Everyone

About a year ago I came upon an intriguing article in the UK *Independent* with the provocative title "Glaxo chief: Our drugs do not work on most patients."[12] It attributes the following to GlaxoSmithKline's chief geneticist, Dr. Allen Roses: " 'The vast majority of drugs—more than 90 per cent—only work in 30 or 50 per cent of the people,' Dr. Roses said. 'I wouldn't say that most drugs don't work. I would say that most drugs work in 30 to 50 per cent of people.

---

[12]Connor, S. Glaxo chief: Our drugs do not work on most patients. *The Independent*, December 8, 2003. Available at http://www.independent.co.uk/news/science/glaxo-chief-our-drugs-do-not-work-on-most-patients-575942.html

Drugs out there on the market work, but they don't work in everybody.' "

In essence, what Dr. Roses was referring to is the phenomenon of *heterogeneous treatment effect* (HTE), described aptly by David Kent and colleagues as the fact that "the effectiveness and safety of a treatment varies across the patient population." The authors preface it by saying that, although evidence-based medicine has enjoyed broad acceptance among developers of guidelines and recommendations, there are reasons to be concerned that the results of population data do not shed enough light on the office encounter, where the patient's individual physiology, values, and wishes may run counter to that group experience. The authors by no means advocate a return to opinion-based medicine. Instead they call for a better understanding of "how the effectiveness and safety of a treatment varies [sic] across the patient population (referred to as heterogeneity of treatment effect [HTE]) so as to make optimal decisions for each patient."[13]

So don't worry: When someone brings an evidence-based guideline to you and insists that, unless you comply 95% of the time, you are providing less than great quality of care and you say, "This guideline does

---

[13]Kent, D. M., Rothwell, P. M., Ioannidis, J. P. A., Altman, D. G., & Hayward, R. A. Assessing and reporting heterogeneity in treatment effects in clinical trials: A proposal. *Trials* 2010; 11:85. Available at http://www.trialsjournal.com/content/11/1/85

not represent my patients," you are actually not crazy. To be sure, a good evidence-based practice guideline will apply to *most* patients encountered with a particular condition. But the devil, of course, is in the details. As I pointed out in the previous chapter, we impose statistical principles onto data to whip them into submission. When we do a good job, we acknowledge the limitations of what is provided to us by measures of central tendency. But so much of the time I see physicians relying on such flawed measures of statistical significance as just the p value (we will wax poetic about it at length in Chapter 20 of the book) to compare the effects that I am forced to conclude that the variation around the center is mostly lost on us. And further, how does this variance help a clinician faced with an individual patient who has at best a probability of response on some continuum of a population of probabilities? And more important, how will this individual patient view his risk/benefit balance for a particular therapy through the prism of his own values?

I hope it is clear how important it is to examine the data that have gone into a recommendation: What is the degree of HTE in the studies, and, specifically, what is known about the population that your patient represents? The less HTE and the more knowledge about specific subgroups, the more confident you can be in how the therapy will work in the office. Ultimately, however, each patient is a universe onto herself, since no two people will share the same genetics, environmental exposures, chronic condition profile, or other treatments, to name just a few potential characteristics that may impact response to therapy.

This is why we need better trials, trials where people are represented more broadly, leading to an increase in external validity. To make this information useful at the bedside, we need a priori plans to analyze many different subgroups, as that will give clinicians at least some granularity so desperately needed in the office.

Until technology gives us a better way (assuming that it will), a systematic approach to treatment trials should be undertaken where possible. N of 1 trials, though not appropriate in every situation, may be quite helpful in optimizing treatment in some chronic conditions. These trials are exactly what they sound like and are appropriate for the office setting when the condition in question is chronic. In these pragmatic studies the patient is cycled through a treatment, alternating with a placebo or another treatment, in a blinded fashion. Although some infrastructure is needed, with the advent of health information technologies, these trials may become less daunting and, in aggregate, provide some very useful and generalizable information on what happens in the real world. Each clinician will need to take some ownership in advancing our collective understanding of the diseases she/he treats. This may truly be the disruptive innovation we are all looking for to improve the quality of care and to promote better health and quality of life.

CHAPTER 8

When the Brain Gets in the Way, Part 1[14]

This chapter and the one that follows are intended to review some of the evidence for how we interpret scientific data. When we examine any study, there are several questions that we ask before we even engage in incorporating its results into our mental database on the subject, as we will address in detail in Part Two of this book. Briefly, once we have determined that the study asks a valid and important question, we focus on the methods. It is here that we talk about threats to

---

[14]Unless otherwise noted, all material in this chapter refers to: Kaptchuk, T. J. Effect of interpretive bias on research evidence. *BMJ* 2003; 326:1453. Reprinted by permission of BMJ Publishing Group Ltd.

validity, of which the traditional quartet consists of (1) bias, (2) confounding, (3) misclassification, and (4) generalizability. These are the tangible pitfalls in which we bog down when evaluating studies. But there are other, more insidious sources of bias. So nefarious are they that we work hard to convince ourselves that we are not subject to them (but, of course, our colleagues are).

Ted Kaptchuk at Harvard has done work in this area. A few words about Ted: If you look him up, his credentials come up as ODM, which stands for Oriental Doctor of Medicine. He did his ODM studies in a five–year Oriental Medicine program in China. If this very fact discredits all of his work for you, dear reader, you are then a perfect example of some of the cognitive biases that he describes. So, if you can bring yourself to keep reading, you might get a greater insight into your aversion to some ideas, a reaction perhaps not quite as rational as you think.

Dr. Kaptchuk published a paper in 2003, which summarizes several pervasive cognitive traps that, while at times working in our favor, frequently steer us away from potentially valid scientific conclusions. The first type of cognitive bias he addresses is called "interpretation" bias. The opening paragraph of the paper sets the stage:

Facts do not accumulate on the blank slates of researchers' minds, and data simply do not speak for themselves. Good science inevitably embodies a tension between the empiricism of concrete data and the rationalism of deeply held convictions. Unbiased interpretation of data is as important as performing rigorous experiments. This evaluative process is never totally objective or completely independent of scientists' convictions or theoretical apparatus. This article elaborates on an insight of Vandenbroucke, who noted that "facts and theories remain inextricably linked. . . . At the cutting edge of scientific progress, where new ideas develop, we will never escape subjectivity." Interpretation can produce sound judgments or systematic error. Only hindsight will enable us to tell which has occurred. Nevertheless, awareness of the systematic errors that can occur in evaluative processes may facilitate the self regulating forces of science and help produce reliable knowledge sooner rather than later.

The idea that evidence accumulation tends to be unidirectional is something that I have explored in my own writing:

The scientific community, based on some statistical and other methodological considerations, has come to a consensus around what constitutes valid study designs. This consensus is based on a profound understanding of the tools available to us to answer the questions at hand. The key concept here is that of "available tools." As new tools become available, we introduce them into our research armamentarium to go deeper and further. What we need to appreciate, however, is that "deeper" and "further" are directional words: They imply the same direction as before, only beyond the current stopping point. This is a natural way for us to think, since even our tools are built on the foundation of what has been used previously.[15]

Kaptchuk goes on to point out that we do not often burden ourselves with identifying cognitive biases and that this happens simply because we don't know how to measure what happens at the nexus of data and judgment. As you will note in Part Two of this book, when we focus our attention on threats to validity in general and on bias in particular, we focus on the cold technical aspects of studies and their analyses, rather than on the much more nebulous and elusive mind traps that afflict both the investigator and the reader alike.

Indeed, the impact of our preconceived notions on

---

[15]Zilberberg, M. D. Evidence: *What* the bleep do we really know? *Healthcare, etc.* weblog. April 6, 2010. Available at http://evimedgroup.blogspot.com/2010/04/evidence-what-bleep-do-we-really-know.html

how we interpret and assimilate new data is essentially ignored because we do not have a good way to measure it. We just know that it is there.

Then there is the relationship between quality assessment of a study and "confirmation" bias. What underlies confirmation bias is our own preconceived notions of what is correct. In other words, we are likely to scrutinize more thoroughly the results that disagree with our understanding of the subject than those that agree with it. And this is not always wrong. Evidence that diverges radically from the current understanding of a phenomenon should be viewed skeptically, lest we be led astray by a chance finding. However, this bias rears its ugly head whenever we happen to hold a differing viewpoint and often prevents us from examining the data objectively.

Does this sound familiar? Remember the recently recommended changes to mammography screening from the US Preventive Services Task Force? How about when the news of the WHI results about hormone replacement therapy became public? I will not belabor either, as much is available on this from other sources. Suffice it to say that virtually all of the cognitive biases described in Kaptchuk's paper were at play. We are simply more likely to poke holes in and to reject anything that disagrees with what we think we know. This is one of the difficulties in advancing scientific knowledge, since all of us are far more skeptical of what contradicts than of what confirms our beliefs.

How many of us have found ourselves saying "I do not believe these data" because they have contradicted our previously held notions? And how often do we nod vigorously and agree with the data that agree with us? To deny this is simply disingenuous. And if this is too anecdotal for you, there is experimental evidence that confirms this:

> Two examples might be helpful. Koehler asked 297 advanced university science graduate students to evaluate two supposedly genuine experiments after being induced with different "doses" of positive and negative beliefs through false background papers. Questionnaires showed that their beliefs were successfully manipulated. The students gave significantly higher rating to reports that agreed with their manipulated beliefs, and the effect was greater among those induced to hold stronger beliefs. In another experiment, 398 researchers who had previously reviewed experiments for a respected journal were unknowingly randomly assigned to assess fictitious reports of treatment for obesity. The reports were identical except for the description of the intervention being tested. One intervention was an unproved but credible treatment (hydroxycitrate); the other was an implausible treatment (homoeopathic sulphur). Quality assessments were significantly higher for the more plausible version.

The next two related cognitive biases examined in the context of expectation of a result are called "rescue" and "auxiliary hypothesis" biases. Rescue bias is somewhat similar to confirmation bias. The difference lies in the fact that whereas confirmation bias is not deliberate, the rescue bias is frequently a willful attempt to discredit the evidence that contradicts our convictions.

One classic example of the rescue and auxiliary hypothesis biases cited by Kaptchuk was the letters to the editor generated by a vintage study in the 1970s that showed that a coronary artery bypass was no better than medical treatment among veterans in a randomized controlled trial. The endpoint of the trial was one that we can be most certain of: death. And here is what is particularly telling about these biases in these debates. The supporters of bypass found flaws in the study design that would steer the conclusions away from effectiveness of the surgery. At the same time, its detractors extolled the virtues of the design that supported their point of view.

Echoes of the recent mammography debate come through loud and clear. And from these fiercely held views springs an additional and related cognitive bias: the auxiliary hypothesis bias. It is characterized by mental contortions that we go through to come up with a set of different experimental conditions that would have resulted in a different outcome, one held dear by us. And this is exactly what is still happening in the menopausal hormone replacement therapy world, where the mammoth WHI-HRT randomized controlled trial put its use in serious question. Yet HRT's committed proponents continue to argue that the population wasn't the right age, the dose and composition of the therapy were wrong, and so on and so forth, all the while fitting into the structure of the auxiliary hypothesis bias. And mind you, all of these hypotheses may be worth exploring; but my bet is that had the trial results conformed to their prior expectations, the scrutiny of the design would be orders of magnitude weaker.

To summarize, here are the cognitive biases we have discussed so far:

1. *Interpretation bias:* Our interpretation of the validity of data relies upon our own preconceived judgments and notions of the field.
2. *Confirmation bias:* We tend to be less skeptical and therefore less critical of a study that supports than one that goes against what we think we know and understand.
3. *Rescue bias:* When a study does not conform to our preconceived ideas, we tend to find selective faults with the study in order to rescue our notions.
4. *Auxiliary hypothesis bias:* It is the "wrong patient population and wrong dose" bias.

The next chapter rounds out our discussion with "plausibility" (or "mechanism"), "time will tell," and "hypothesis and orientation" biases.

CHAPTER 9

When the Brain Gets in the Way, Part 2[16]

A s if it were not enough that we will defend our preconceived notions tooth and nail, make up stories
for why they may have been refuted, and maintain that
a different design would fix the universe, as we saw in
the previous chapter, we also fall prey to the three remaining types of bias that Kaptchuk talks about in his
paper: (1) plausibility (or mechanism), (2) time will tell,
and (3) hypothesis and orientation.

---

[16]Unless otherwise noted, all material in this chapter refers to:
Kaptchuk, T. J. Effect of interpretive bias on research evidence.
BMJ 2003; 326:1453 Reprinted by permission of BMJ Publish-
ing Group Ltd.

The so-called "plausibility" or "mechanism" bias, simply put, means that "evidence is more easily accepted when supported by accepted scientific mechanisms." I fear that I cannot improve on the examples that Dr. Kaptchuk cites in his paper:

> For example, the early negative evidence for hormone replacement therapy would have undoubtedly been judged less cautiously if a biological rationale had not already created a strong expectation that oestrogens would benefit the cardiovascular system. Similarly, the rationale for antiarrhythmic drugs for myocardial infarction was so imbedded that each of three antiarrhythmic drugs had to be proved harmful individually before each trial could be terminated. And the link between *Helicobacter pylori* and peptic ulcer was rejected initially because the stomach was considered to be too acidic to support bacterial growth.

Of course, this is how science continues on its evolutionary path. And, of course, we as scientists are first to acknowledge this fact. And while this is true and we should certainly be saluted for this forthright admission and willingness to be corrected, the trouble is that this tendency does not become clear until it can be visualized through the 20/20 lens of the retrospectoscope. When we are in the midst of our debates, we frequently cite biologic plausibility or our current understanding of underlying mechanisms as a barrier to accepting not just a divergent result but even a new hypothesis. So entrenched are we in this type of thinking that we feel scientifically justified to disparage anything without an apparent, plausible, mechanistic explanation. And Dr. Kaptchuk's examples provide evidence that at least some of the time we will have to get used to how we look with egg on our faces. Of course, the trouble is that we cannot prospectively know what will be wheat and what will be chaff. My preferred way of dealing with this uncertainty, one of many, is just to acknowledge the possibility. To do otherwise seems arrogant.

Next comes the colorfully named "time will tell" bias. This refers to the different thresholds for the amount of evidence we have for accepting something as valid. This in and of itself would not seem all that objectionable if it were not for a couple of features. The first is the feature of extremes. An "evangelist" jumps on the bandwagon of the data as soon as it is out. The only issue here is that an evangelist may have a conflict of interest, be it financial, professional, or intellectual, where there is some vested interest in the data. One of these vested interests, the intellectual, is very difficult to detect and to measure, to the point that many peer-review journals do not even require us to disclose whether a potential for it exists. Yet, how can it not, when we build our careers on moving in a particular direction of research (another illustration of its unidirectionality) and when our entire professional, and occasionally personal, selves may be invested in proving it right? At the other extreme is the naysayer who needs large heaps of supporting data before accepting the evidence. And here as well, the same conflicts of interest abound, but in the direction away from what is being shown. To illustrate this, Kaptchuk gives one of my favorite quotes from Max Planck: "A new scientific truth does not triumph by convincing its opponents and making them see the light, but rather because its opponents eventually die, and a new generation grows up that is familiar with it."

The final bias is "hypothesis and orientation" bias, in which the researcher's bias in the hypothesis affects how data are gathered in the study. The infamous placebo effect fits nicely into this category, where, if not blinded to experimental conditions, we tend to see effects that we want to see. You would think that blinding would alleviate this type of a bias, yet, as Kaptchuk cites, even when blinded, RCTs, for example, sponsored by pharmaceutical companies are more likely to be positive than those that are not. To be fair (and Kaptchuk is), the anatomy of this discrepancy is not well understood. As he mentions, this may have something to do with a publication bias, where negative trials do not come to publication either because of methodological flaws or because of suppression of (or sometimes, with less malfeasance, even due to apathy about) negative data.

I cannot help but bring up Dr. Kaptchuk's latest discovery, however. Back in December of 2010 he and his colleagues published a study that startled the world.[17] In this RCT they compared "open-label" placebos to no treatment in the setting of irritable bowel syndrome. And contrary to expectation, the group receiving this open-label placebo did better than the control group who received no treatment. What this result implies is that, at least for some ailments, giving placebo with the full knowledge of the patient can still have therapeutic efficacy! How does this work, and what does it say about our cognitive biases? Ed Yong, a science writer and blogger at *Discover Magazine,* put it this way: "Kaptchuk himself says, 'I suspect that just performing "the ritual of medicine" could have activated or primed self-healing mechanisms.'"[18]

There is always more to say about this complex subject, but we have to stop somewhere. And lest we walk away tormented by this purgatory of uncertainty, I will

---

[17]Kaptchuk, T. J., Friedlander, E., Kelley, J. M., Sanchez, M. N., Kokkotou, E., et al. Placebos Without Deception: A Randomized Controlled Trial in Irritable Bowel Syndrome. *PLoS ONE* 2010; 5:e15591

[18]Yong, E. Evidence that placebos could work even if you tell people they're taking placebos, in *Not Exactly Rocket Science* Blog, *Discover Magazine*, December 22, 2010. Available at http://blogs.discovermagazine.com/notrocketscience/2010/12/22/evidence-that-placebos-could-work-even-if-you-tell-people-they%E2%80%99re-taking-placebos/

let Dr. Kaptchuk's final paragraph be the hopeful conclusion: "Ultimately, brute data are coercive. However, a view that science is totally objective is mythical, and ignores the human element of medical inquiry. Awareness of subjectivity will make assessment of evidence more honest, rational, and reasonable."

CHAPTER 10

The Beautiful Uncertainty of Science

Polarized and polarizing discussions are the purview of politics, not science. As in other venues, we only get further away from the truth, if such a thing exists, by retreating into our cognitive corners. These corners are comfortable places, with our comrades-in-arms sharing our passionate opinions. Yet this is not the way to get to a better understanding.

Because I spend so much time contemplating our larger understanding of science, Felicity Barringer's post titled "Are We Hard-Wired to Doubt Science?" on the *New York Times* "Green" blog proved to be a really inflammatory way to suck me into thinking about everything I am interested in integrating: scientific method, science literacy and communication, and brain science.[19] The author, on the heels of doing a story on the opposition to smart meters (smart meters are wireless electricity meters, and there is opposition to them due to concerns about their potential health effects) in California, was led to try to understand why we are so quick to reject science: "But some very intelligent people I interviewed had little use for the existing (if sparse) science. How, in a rational society, does one understand those who reject science, a common touchstone of what is real and verifiable?" She asks reasonably how it is that people remain wedded to their beliefs, such as that vaccines cause autism or, conversely, that human activity is not responsible for climate change, despite mountains of scientific evidence to the contrary.

Barringer argues that, in essence, new data are unable to sway our opinion because of rescue bias, or our drive to preserve what we think we know to be true and to reject what our intuition tells us is false. If we follow this argument to its logical conclusion, it means that we should just throw our hands up in the air and accept the status quo, whatever it is. That is not so: We need to come to a better understanding.

---

[19]Barringer F. Are We Hard-Wired to Doubt Science? *Green, A Blog About Energy and the Environment. New York Times*, accessed February 1, 2011. Available at http://green.blogs .nytimes.com/2011/02/01/are-we-hard-wired-to-doubt-science/ ?partner=rss&emc=rss#preview

Everyone needs to understand what science is and, even more important, what it is not. First, science is not dogma. Karl Popper had a very simple litmus test for scientific thinking: He asked how you would go about disproving a particular idea. If you think that the idea is above being disproved, then you are engaging in dogma and not science. The essence of scientific method is developing a hypothesis either from a systematically observed pattern or from a theoretical model. The hypothesis is necessarily formulated as the null, making the assumption of "no association" the departure point for proving the contrary. So, to "prove" that the association is present, you need to rule out any other potential explanation for what may appear to be an association. For example, if thunder were always followed by rain, it might be easy to engage in a *post hoc ergo propter hoc* fallacy and to conclude that thunder caused rain. But before this could become a scientific theory, you would have to show that, after a thorough search, no other cause for rain could be found.

So the point is that science is driven by postulating the null hypothesis and then disproving it. It is only feasible to disprove a hypothesis if (1) the association exists and (2) the constellation of phenomena is not explained by something else. And here is the next and critical point, the point that produces equal parts frustration and inspiration to learn more: That "something else" as the explanation for a certain association is by definition informed only by what we know today. It is this very quality of knowledge production, the constancy of the pursuit, that lends the only certain property to science: the property of uncertainty. And our brains have a hard time holding and living with this uncertainty.

The tension between uncertainty and the need to make public policy has taken on a political life of its own. What started out as a modest storm of subversion of science by politics in the tobacco debate has now escalated into a cyclone of everyday leveraging of the scientific uncertainties for political and economic gains. After all, how can we balance the accounting between the theoretical models predicting climate doom in the future and the robust current-day economic gains produced by the very pollution that feeds these models? How can we even conceive that our food production system, yielding more abundant and cheaper food than ever before, is driving the epidemic of obesity and the catastrophe of antimicrobial resistance? And because we are talking about science, and because, as that populist philosopher Yogi Berra famously quipped, "Predictions are hard, especially about the future," the uncertainty of our estimates overshadows the probability of their correctness. Yet by the time the future becomes the present, we will be faced with potentially insurmountable challenges of a new world.

I have heard some scientists express reluctance about "coming clean" to the public about just how uncertain our knowledge is. Nonsense! What we need is greater transparency, public literacy, and engagement. Science is not something that happens in the bastions of higher education or behind the thick walls of corporations. Science is all around and within us. The language of science may seem daunting, but it should not make you afraid—patterns of a language are easy to decipher with some willingness and a dictionary. Our brains are attuned to the most beautiful explanations of the universe. And science is what provides these explanations.

Self-determination is predicated upon knowledge and understanding. Abdicating our ability to understand the scientific method leaves us subject to political demagoguery. Don't be a puppet. We are all born scientists. Embrace your curiosity. Tune out the noise of those at the margins who are not willing to engage in a sensible dialogue; leave them to their schoolyard brawling. Start learning the basics of scientific philosophy and thought. Allow the uncertainty of knowledge to excite and delight you. You will not be disappointed.

CHAPTER 11

In Praise of Not Knowing

Recently I had the occasion to tell my children an old secret: Until I was into my forties, I had a strong belief that the rest of the people in the world knew something I did not know. I don't mean just about stuff I really don't know, but about everything! It was unnerving, anxiety provoking, and self-defeating. Then one day I had the epiphany that most humans feel this way, not just me. So, we should be humbled by not knowing and move on.

Even more recently this line of self-examination has led me to the conclusion that I end up saying "I don't know" a lot. I read a definitive tweet from someone I respect, and I say to myself "I don't know"; I read a new paper in a journal and say, "Gee, I don't know"; I hear a political speech, and I walk away saying, "I just don't know." Is it that I am an idiot or intellectually lazy? Perhaps. But what is occurring to me more and more lately is that what we are convinced of today will be much less certain and obvious tomorrow, barring some truly sacred cows. This is called growth; and as far as I can tell, it is a desirable development.

Yet saying "I don't know" sometimes means that it just does not make sense to take sides. I do know that we have to apply current knowledge and not wait for perfect information, but I still don't see the need to get polarized: Most of the time we act like there are only two possibilities and they are diametrically opposed to one another. Well, these are false dichotomies, which may be an unintended consequence of our educational system, drilling into us the idea that there are only two answers to any question: the right one and the wrong one. What if this is not true? What if we change the way we think about the world and, instead of seeing only the black and the white, the left and the right, the correct and the incorrect, we start really seeing the entire continuum of possibilities? We just might stumble on a fantastic variety of solutions to our perennial questions!

A nice mind experiment could be trying to think without using words. Can we do that? It is thoroughly difficult, since it is language that seems to bracket our conceptual understanding of the world within and around us. Take the words *race* and *gender*, for example. These are human-made and -defined terms, which are meant to distinguish rather than blur. Despite these being made-up ideas, just think how uncomfortable a person with an ambiguous gender identity can make us. Why? Because she/he does not fit into our preconceived dichotomy. Uncertainty is uncomfortable, and dichotomies cure uncertainty. But I am not sure that nature is all that into dichotomies.

The human brain is wired for "belonging." I believe it is for this reason that we gravitate to our respective extreme corners of thinking and being instead of meeting somewhere in the aisle. The aisle is an uncomfortable place, yet that is where we must aim to be. All the borders we have created are imaginary separations. Instead we can reposition them as the glue that unifies what lies to either side.

Here is to more not knowing!

CHAPTER 12

A Constructive Way to Deal with Uncertainty

When anything is possible, nothing is probable. When a headache is just as likely to be a brain tumor as a sinus or muscle tension problem, every possibility requires equal attention. Remember when we talked about what happens when a screening test is applied to a population at a low risk for the disease being screened (see Chapters 3 and 4)? Positive results become overwhelmingly false, and the diagnostic tail-chasing that ensues not only wastes time and resources but also results in some dire adverse consequences. Recall the story that I told of the woman who had to undergo a heart transplant after a procedure that followed up a false positive test resulted in a catastrophic complication. In fact, it is this indiscriminate search for the possible that has landed us in the mess that we call our twenty-first-century healthcare. Here is what I mean.

When a person goes to his doctor with a problem that needs to "get fixed," a pivotal triad of presentation-diagnosis-treatment ensues. The three steps are as follows:

1. **History, physical examination, and a differential diagnosis**
   When the patient shows up with a complaint, a constellation of symptoms and signs, a good clinician collects this information and funnels it through a mesh of possibilities, ruling certain conditions in and others out to derive the initial differential diagnosis.

2. **Diagnostic testing**
   Having gone through the exercise in step 1, the practitioner then decides on appropriate diagnostic testing in order to narrow down further the possible reasons for the person's state.

3. **Treatment**
   Finally, having reviewed all the data, the clinician makes the therapeutic choice.

These three steps seem dead simple, and we have all experienced them as patient or clinician or both. Yet the cause for the current catastrophic state of our healthcare system lies within the brackets of each of these three little domains.

The cause is our failure to *acknowledge* the vast universe of uncertainty that is dotted sparsely with the galaxies of definiteness, all shrouded in false confidence. And while the cause and the way to address it are conceptually simple, the remedy is not easy to implement.

Let's examine what goes on in step 1, the compilation of history and physical to generate a differential diagnosis. This is usually an implicit process that takes place mostly at a subconscious level, where the mind makes connections between the current patient and what the clinician has learned and experienced. What does that mean? It means that the clinician, within the constraints of the ever-shrinking appointment, has to listen, examine, elicit, and put together all of the data in such a way as to cram them into a few little diagnostic boxes, many of which contain much more material than a human brain can hold all at once. And this is true even if that brain happens to be above average in human cognition. What overtakes at this step is a bunch of heuristics and biases. *Heuristics* are mental shortcuts that can serve us well, but they can also lead us astray, particularly under conditions of extreme uncertainty, as in a healthcare encounter. As for cognitive biases, just check out Chapters 8 and 9 devoted to them.

The picture that emerges at this step is one of fragments of gathered information being fit into fragments of studies and experience, stirred with mental short-cuts, and poured into a bunch of baking tins shaped like specific diagnoses. Is there any room in this process for assigning objective probabilities to any of these events? Well, there is an illusion of doing so; but even this step is done by feel, rather than by computation. So while there is some awareness of a probabilistic hierarchy, it is more chaos than science. Given this picture, it's a wonder it actually works as well as it does.

The next step in this recipe is the diagnostic workup. What ensues here is utter Wild West, particularly as new technologies are adopted at breakneck speed without any thought to the interpretation of data that they are capable of spitting out. Here the confusion of the first step gets magnified exponentially, just as it seduces us into further illusion of certainty. The uncertainties in arriving at the differential get multiplied by the imperfections of diagnostic tests to give the encounter truly quantum properties: You may know the results or you may know the patient, but you may not know both at the same time. No test is perfect; and because of this simple truth, unless we know the pre-test probability of the disease in a particular patient, as well as the characteristics of the test, we have no idea about the context of these results. Taking them at face value is a grave error.

What follows these results are frequently more diagnostic hits or misses, as the likelihood of harm and escalating expenditures without any added value rises.

Then comes the treatment, with its many uncertainties and the potential for adverse events. So, what's to be done?

I think that there is a simple solution to this, and in its simplicity it will be characteristically difficult to implement: education. And I don't just mean medical education. Everything about which I have talked in this chapter echoes back to the concept of probability. In secondary education, by the time a student becomes eligible to study it, she has been made to feel that she does not have the facility for math and that, furthermore, math is boring and useless. So the percentage of kids who leave high school having been exposed to some study of probability is woefully small. And those who do get exposure to it walk out of class perfectly able to bet on a game of craps or a horse race but without a clue how to apply these ideas to the world in which they live.

If you are dubious that physicians are just like the rest of the world when it comes to interpreting probability, let me tell you about a study that was done back in the 1970s.[20] The study was conducted in one of the hospitals affiliated with Harvard Medical School in Boston. The investigators posed a simple problem to 60 physicians and physicians-in-training: "If a test to

---

[20]Casscells, W., Schoenberger, A., & Graboys, T. B. Interpretation by physicians of clinical laboratory results. *New England Journal of Medicine* 1978; 299:999–1001

detect a disease whose prevalence is 1/1000 has a false positive rate of 5 per cent, what is the chance that a person found to have a positive result actually has the disease, assuming that you know nothing about the person's symptoms or signs?" To answer this question, all you need to do is set up a table similar to the ones we utilized in Chapters 3 and 4. If you do that, you arrive at the startling answer 2%. This means that 98 out of 100 positive tests are actually false positive. In the study only a small proportion, 18%, of the doctors and doctors-in-training arrived at the correct answer. Most disturbing, however, was the fact that nearly half of these eminent responders, 27 out of 60, arrived at the figure of 95% as indicating true positives, or presence of the disease. And it is this 93% gap that serves as the pool for overdiagnosis and overtreatement.

So the study makes it clear that both those who progress into healthcare and those who don't have heard the word *probability* but cannot quite understand how it impacts them beyond their chance of winning the lottery. And unfortunately, I have to tell you that if I relied on what I learned in medical school about probability, well, let's just say it is highly improbable that I would be writing this right now.

But the education that I am advocating takes time, and many people are plain afraid of probability. What can we do to remedy the situation in the short term? The answer is that we already manage uncertainty in other areas of our lives all the time. We consider the odds of rain when choosing what to wear. We do (or at least we should do) a quick mental risk-benefit analysis before buying a burger at Quickie-Mart. We choose our driving routes to work based on the probability of encountering heavy traffic. We do this mental calculus subconsciously but reliably, mostly getting it right. What is odd, though, is that we operate under a misapprehension that medicine is devoid of uncertainty. Bollocks! The only certain thing about medicine is uncertainty. As I have shown, this uncertainty gets magnified in the office encounter.

So, what is the immediate solution? It is simple: We all need to learn what questions to ask of our doctors and other healthcare providers. Instead of nodding our heads vigorously to everything our doctors say, we should put up our hands and ask how certain she/he is that she/he is on the right track. Here are a dozen questions to help start this conversation:

1. What are the odds that we have the diagnosis wrong?
2. What are the odds that the test you are ordering will give us the right answer, given the odds of my having the condition that you are testing me for?
3. How are we going to interpret results that are equivocal?
4. What follow-up testing will need to happen if the results are equivocal?

5. What are the implications of further testing in terms of diagnostic certainty and invasiveness of follow-up testing?

6. If I need an invasive test, what are the odds that it will yield a useful diagnosis that will alter my care?

7. If I need an invasive test, what are the odds of an adverse event, such as infection, bleeding, or even death?

8. What are the odds of missing something deadly if we forgo this diagnostic testing?

9. What are the odds that the treatment you are prescribing for this condition will improve the condition?

10. How much improvement can I expect with this treatment, if there is to be improvement?

11. What are the odds that I will have an adverse event related to this treatment, and what are the odds of a serious adverse event that may land me in a hospital, or even such as death?

12. How much will all of this cost in the context of the benefit I am likely to derive from it?

And in the end, we need to understand where these odds are coming from—the clinician's gut or hard data or both? I prefer it when the clinician integrates both, which, I believe, was the original intent of evidence-based medicine.

Perhaps for some of us, this is a stretch: We don't like

numbers, we are intimidated by the setting, the doc may be unhappy with the interrogation. But it is truly incumbent on all of us to accept the responsibility for sharing in these clinical decisions. I believe that clinicians today are much more in tune with shared decision making and understand the value of participatory medicine. And if they are not, educate them. Ultimately, it is your own attitude toward risk, and not just the naked data combined with the clinician's perceptions of your attitude, that should drive all of these decisions.

Knowledge is empowering, and empowerment is good for everyone, patient and clinician alike. As patients, taking control of what happens to us in a medical encounter can only bring higher odds of a desirable outcome. For physicians, a cogent conversation about their recommendations may help safeguard against future litigation, not to mention augment the satisfaction in the relationship. And, thus, starting to discuss probabilities explicitly is very likely to get us to a better place in terms of both quality and costs of medical care. And in the process it may very well train us in how to make better decisions in the rest of our lives.

Here is a summary: First, we need to acknowledge the colossal uncertainties in medicine. Once we have done so, we need to understand that such uncertainties require a probabilistic approach in order to optimize care. Finally, such probabilistic approach has to be taught early and often. All of us, clinicians and patients alike, are responsible for creating this monster that we call healthcare in the twenty-first century. We will not train the monster to behave by adding more parts. The only way to train it is to train our brains to be much more critical and to engage in a conversation about probabilities. Without this shift a constructive change in how medicine is done in this country is, well, improbable.

PART TWO

Evaluation

NOW THAT WE ARE AWARE of the elements that make scientific ideas a moving target, we can delve into some concrete ways of evaluating studies that provide evidence that feeds everyday decisions in medicine. Many of the categories of study evaluation I discuss in this book originated from "Primers" available from the American College of Physicians in their *Effective Clinical Practice* series.[21] Over the years that I have been reading medical literature, doing clinical research, and writing, however, I have developed my own under-

---

[21]American College of Physicians. Primers. Effective Clinical Practice. Available at http://www.acponline.org/clinical_information/journals_publications/ecp/primers.htm

standing and approaches that broadly fit into these categories. What you will see in the next chapters is the result of these years of thinking and refining ideas.

CHAPTER 13

The Study Question

Let's start at the beginning. Why do we do research and write papers? No, not just to get famous, tenured, or funded. The fundamental task of science is to formulate and answer questions. The big questions of all time get broken down into manageable chunks that can be answered with experimental or observational scientific methods. The manageable chunks in the medical sciences are usually constructed by asking narrowly what the impact of a small and specific alteration to the system is, be it disease, drug, procedure, or an environmental exposure, for example. Implicit in this formulation is a comparison: specific alteration present vs. specific alteration absent. This is why we talk about our studies having controls. While the experimental condition is that of the alteration of interest being present, the control represents circumstances similar in all ways with the exception of the alteration of interest. We refer to this particular alteration of interest as "exposure." The answers to these manageable chunks integrated together provide the model for the universe as we understand it.

Along these lines, there are primary and secondary research studies. The primary studies report on individual investigations and serve as the subject of this section of the book. In contrast, secondary studies usually represent a reworking or a synthesis of what has been published as primary data. Meta-analysis is an example of secondary studies.

Clearly, the question is the most important part of the equation, and this is why in my semester-long graduate epidemiology course on the evaluative sciences we spend fully the first four to five weeks talking about how to develop a valid and answerable question. The scientific method, as articulated by the philosopher Karl Popper, relies on developing hypotheses that are inherently falsifiable. Unless and until hypotheses are disproved, we rely on them as models for how things work. In the pragmatic domain of clinical science, where our results may almost immediately benefit or harm patient care, the importance of the question posed demands particular scrutiny. In other words, what is the use of a valid question or hypothesis if it does not shed any light on some important aspect of the practice of medicine? Hence, the first consideration that we address is this: Is the study question important?

This is a bit of a loaded question, though. Important to whom? How is *important* defined? This is somewhat opaque, yet it requires a discussion. In clinical research, an important question is one that may touch many patients, such as what is the risk-benefit balance of HRT in preventing coronary heart disease among menopausal women? In the context of an individual patient, both for that patient and for her clinician in the office with her, however, the question may become: Is the study question important to me/my patient? So, importance is dependent on perspective. Nevertheless, there are questions on whose validity we can all agree. For example, how does our current fast-food life style promote obesity and diabetes?

Regardless of how we feel about the importance of the question, we must first identify it, and it is impossible to talk about identifying anything without first understanding the geography of a scientific paper. At the beginning of a scientific paper, you will frequently see an *abstract*, or a brief summary of the report. Most of the time, the journals require what is called a "structured" abstract. This means that the authors need to break it up into several sections, usually including an Introduction or a Background, followed by Methods, Results, and Conclusions. Although there are some variations on this structure, all of the content reflects these divisions and echoes back to the structure of the body of the paper. If you look at the WHI-HRT paper, you will see slightly different headings, though all of them can be mapped back to the four that I mentioned. Thus, Context and Objectives are Background; Design, Interventions, and Main Outcomes and Measures fall into the general Methods category; and Results and Conclusions are precisely that. What follows the abstract keeps closely to these specifications as well, save for an additional section called Discussion, where the authors can highlight the important parts of their findings and put them in perspective, given what is already known about the topic.

Now that we understand our way around the paper, back to the question. You usually find it buried in the last paragraph of the Introduction section, and this is borne out in the WHI-HRT: "The WHI is the first randomized trial to directly address whether estrogen plus progestin has a favorable or unfavorable effect on CHD incidence and on overall risks and benefits in predominantly healthy women." [22]

Most of the questions we ask relate to etiologic relationships (*etiology* simply means "cause"). There are three simple criteria that need to be met for a causal relationship to be likely:

---

[22]Writing group for the Women's Health Initiative Investigators. Risks and Benefits of Estrogen Plus Progestin in Healthy Postmenopausal Women: Principal Results from the Women's Health Initiative Randomized Controlled Trial. *JAMA* 2002; 288:321–333 Available at http://jama.ama-assn.org/content/288/3/321.full.pdf+html

1. The cause must occur before the effect.
2. The cause and the effect must be statistically related, or correlated.
3. There is no other plausible explanation for the findings.

If you remember these three criteria, you will be well on your way to understanding the implications of research and what certain study designs can and cannot tell us.

You have probably heard many times that an observational study cannot answer a causal question. So why do we bother with the time, energy, and money needed to run observational studies? Without getting too much into the weeds, philosophers of science tell us that no single study design can give us unequivocal evidence of causality. We can merely come close to it. What does this mean in practical terms? It means that, although most observational studies are still interested in causality rather than a mere association, we have to be more circumspect in how we interpret the results from observational studies than from interventional ones. But I am jumping ahead.

Once we have identified and established the importance of the question, we need to evaluate its quality. A question of high quality is

1. Clear
2. Specific
3. Answerable

To continue with our example of WHI-HRT, the question in the last sentence of the Introduction section is fairly clear and answerable, though it needs to be a whole lot more specific. This specificity resides in the Methods section, where the exposures, the outcomes, and the hypothesized relationship between the exposures and the outcomes should be clearly defined. The WHI question contrasts sharply with the one I posed earlier regarding fast food and obesity, which possesses none of the three characteristics. It is too broad, and it is open to interpretation. If I were really posing a question in this vein, I would choose a specific population (e.g., adolescent males in the United States) with a single well-defined exposure (e.g., consuming 3 cans of sugar-sweetened soda per day) influencing a single highly specific outcome (e.g., 10% body weight gain) over a predefined period of time (e.g., over 30 weeks). While this is a much narrower question than originally, it is only by answering bundles of such narrow questions and putting the information together that we can arrive at the big picture.

A general principle that I like to teach to my students in the process of formulating their scientific questions is the PICO or PECOT model.[23] In PICO, P = population, I = intervention or exposure, C = comparator, and

---

[23]Sackett, D. L., Richardson, W. S., Rosenberg, W., & Haynes, R. B. (1997). *Evidence-based medicine: How to practice and teach EBM*. New York: Churchill Livingston.

O = outcome. The PECOT model is an adaptation of the PICO for observations over time, resulting in P = population, E = exposure, C = comparator, O = outcome, T = time. These models can help not only to pose the question, but also to unravel the often mysterious and far-from-transparent intent of the investigators.

Let's apply the PECOT model to my obesity question:

P = adolescent males in the United States
E = 3 cans of sugar-sweetened soda per day
C = no sugar-sweetened soda
O = weight gain of 10% of the body weight
T = 30 weeks

Once you have identified the question and dealt with its importance, you are ready to move on to the next step: evaluating the study design as it relates to the question.

CHAPTER 14

Study Design—General Scheme

It is true that the study question should inform the study design. I am sure you are aware of the broadest categorization of study design: observational vs. interventional. When I read a study, after identifying the research question I go through a simple 4–step exercise:

1. I look for what the authors say their study design is. This should be pretty easy to find early in the Methods section of the paper, though that is not always the case.

If it is available,

2. I mentally judge whether or not it is feasible to derive an answer to the posed question using the

current study design. For example, in my work I spend a lot of time thinking about issues of therapeutic effectiveness and cost-effectiveness, and a randomized controlled trial that explores efficacy of a therapy cannot adequately answer the effectiveness questions (I will say more about the difference between efficacy and effectiveness later).

If the design of the study appears appropriate,

3. I structure my reading of the paper in such a way as to verify that the stated design is, in fact, the actual design. If it is, then I move on to evaluate other components of the paper.

If I disagree with the authors about the design,

4. I assign my own understanding to the actual design and go through the same mental list as above with the current understanding in mind. For example, the authors may have called their study a case-control, when in fact the actual design was a cohort. When I notice such discrepancy, I do the rest of my reading with the understanding that it is, contrary to the authors' assertion, a cohort study.

There is a general scheme that is used to categorize study designs (Table 4).

TABLE 4 Common Study Categories and Their Time Frame, Advantages, and Disadvantages[24]

	Time Frame	Advantages	Disadvantages
Interventional			
Randomized controlled trial (RCT)	Prospective	High degree of internal validity	Usually poor generalizability Highly resource intensive
Cross-over	Prospective	Efficient because each subject serves as its own control Increased statistical power	Prolongs study duration May be subject to "carry-over" effect (effect of treatment carries over into control period)
Interrupted time series	Prospective or retrospective	Efficient for implementing quality improvement interventions	Subject to confounding Subject to Hawthorne effect (change is due to being observed rather than due to the intervention)

continued

TABLE 4 (continued)

	Time Frame	Advantages	Disadvantages
Observational			
Ecological	Retrospective	Data easily available	Confounding Ecologic fallacy
Cross-sectional	Snapshot in time	Good for estimating prevalence	Cannot infer causality
Case-control			Can not estimate incidence or prevalence
	Usually retrospective	Efficient when outcome is rare	Susceptible to bias
Cohort	Prospective or retrospective	Good for studying rare, occupational and environmental exposures Good for establishing incidence of the outcome and causality Retrospective are cost-efficient Can have high degree of generalizability	Bias, confounding Prospective are expensive and time-consuming Retrospective rely on available data, and therefore may not have all the relevant data

[24]Based in part on Hulley, S. B., Cummings, S. R., Browner, W. S., Grady, D. G., Hearst, & Newman, T. B. *Designing Clinical Research*, 2nd ed. (Philadelphia, PA: Lippincott Williams & Wilkins, 2001).

As I already mentioned, the first broad division is between observational and interventional studies. An anecdote from my course illustrates that this is not always a straightforward distinction. We were looking at a substudy of the WHI, that pesky undertaking that put in serious question menopausal hormone replacement.[25] The data for this substudy were derived from the three randomized controlled trials (RCT) of (1) hormone replacement, (2) diet, and (3) calcium and vitamin D. The unusual feature was that data from the observational component of the WHI were brought together, or pooled, with the interventional data into one analysis. So, is the current study in question observational or interventional? The answer to this is confusing to the point of pulling the wool over the eyes of even experienced clinicians, as became obvious in the case of my students, all mid-career healthcare professionals.

To answer the question, we need to go back to the definitions of *interventional* and *observational*. To qualify as interventional, a study needs to have the intervention be the deliberate reason for the study. A common example of this type of study is the RCT, the sine qua non of the drug evaluation and approval

---

[25]Neuhouser, M. L., Wassertheil-Smoller, S., Thomson, C., et al. Multivitamin Use and Risk of Cancer and Cardiovascular Disease in the Women's Health Initiative Cohorts. *Archives of Internal Medicine* 2009; 169:294–304

process. Here the drug is administered as the primary study intervention, not as the background of regular treatment. Take a look at the WHI-HRT study, which we have been using as our discussion template. Is it interventional? The answer is "yes," since one of the groups is randomized specifically to drug treatment; and it is this intervention that is the object of the question.

In contrast, an observational study is just that: an opportunistic observation of what is happening to a group of subjects under ordinary circumstances. Here no specific treatment is predetermined by the study design. Given that the study that stumped my students looked at multivitamin supplementation as the main exposure, despite its utilization of the data from RCTs, the study was observational. So, the moral of this tale is to be vigilant and examine the design carefully and thoroughly.

We often hear that observational designs are well suited for hypothesis generation only. Well, this is both true and false. Some observational studies actually can test hypotheses, while others are relegated to generation only. For example, cross-sectional and ecological studies serve to generate hypotheses that must subsequently be tested in another design. To take a recent controversy as an example, the debunked link between vaccinations and autism initially gained steam from the observation that as vaccination rates were rising, so was the incidence of autism. The type of study that uses aggregate data from a group of subjects rather than individual data and shows two events changing at this group or population level either in the same or in the opposite direction is called "ecologic." Similar types of studies gave rise to the vitamin D and cancer association hypothesis, showing geographic variation in cancer rates based on the availability of sun exposure. But, as demonstrated well by the vaccine/autism debacle, running with the links from ecological studies is dangerous because they are prone to a so-called "ecologic fallacy." This occurs when, despite the finding in groups of a linked change of the two factors under investigation, there is absolutely no connection between them at the individual level. So, don't let anyone tell you that they tested a hypothesis in an ecologic study.

Similarly in cross-sectional studies a hypothesis cannot be tested, and, therefore, causation cannot be "proven." This is due to the fundamental property of "a snapshot in time" that defines a cross-sectional study. Since all events in such a study (with few minor exceptions) are measured and, therefore, appear to be happening at the same time, it is not possible to assign causation to the exposure-outcome couplet. These studies, aside from telling us the prevalence of a disease, can merely help us think of further questions to test. An example of a cross-sectional study is the long-standing National Health and Nutrition Examination Survey, often referred to as NHANES. An incredibly ambitious undertaking by the CDC, this series of surveys dealing with public health and nutrition started in the 1960s and continues to this day. One of the most recent findings from this study linked coronary heart disease to exposure to bisphenol A (BPA), a chemical found in some food and water containers, among other places. However, in such a study it is impossible to tell the chicken from the egg: Did people develop heart disease following their exposure to this chemical, or did the exposure follow the onset of heart disease? The only thing that can be said about these results is that there is an association between the two, and this needs to be explored through a different study design, such as a cohort. And incidentally this was recently done by a group in England, who confirmed the link between BPA and heart disease, this time shedding more light on the sequence of events.[26]

So, to connect the design back to the question, if a study purports to "explore a link between exposure X and outcome Y," either an ecologic or a cross-sectional design is okay. But if you see one of these designs used to "test the hypothesis that exposure X causes outcome Y," run the other way screaming.

---

[26]Melzer, D., Osborne, N. J., Henley, W. E., et al. Urinary bisphenol A concentration and risk of future coronary artery disease in apparently healthy men and women. *Circulation 2012*, published online February 21, 2012, as doi:10.1161/ CIRCULATIONAHA.111.069153

CHAPTER 15

Observational Studies

We already addressed two types of observational studies—ecological and cross-sectional—in the previous chapter. Now, let us round out our discussion by describing other observational designs.

Case-control studies are done when the outcome of interest is rare. These are typically retrospective studies, taking advantage of already existing data. Because of this they are quite cost-effective. Cases are defined by the presence of a particular outcome, and controls have to come from a similar underlying population. The exposures are identified backward. One well-known and well-done case-control study questioned the link between cellular telephone use and brain cancer.[27] This outcome, brain cancer, certainly meets the rare outcome criterion and, therefore, is appropriate for this design. In the study, between years 1994 and 1998, 469 patients with brain cancer (cases) were matched to 422 persons without brain cancer (controls); and everyone was interviewed in great detail as to their cellular phone habits. The study found no association between cell phone use and brain cancer, and this might have been for a number of reasons aside from there really being no connection. One major problem, however, with this particular study was the low rates of cellular phone use among both the cases (14%) and the controls (18%).

In all honesty, case-control studies are very tricky to design, analyze, and interpret well. Furthermore, it has been my experience that authors frequently confuse case-control with cohort designs. I cannot tell you how many times as a peer-reviewer I have had to point out to the authors that they have erroneously pegged their study a case-control when in reality it was a cohort. (In the interest of full disclosure, once, many years ago, an editor pointed out a similar error to me in one of my manuscripts.) The hallmark of case-control is that the selection happens at the end of the line, based on the outcome that has occurred, and all other data are collected backward from that point.

Cohort studies define the exposure(s) first and exam-

---

[27]Muskat, J. E., Malkin, M. G., Thompson, S., et al. Handheld Cellular Telephone Use and Risk of Brain Cancer. *JAMA* 2000; 284(23):3001–3007.

ine outcomes that occur following these exposures. Similar to case-control design, retrospective cohort studies are opportunistic in that they look at already collected data (e.g., administrative records, electronic medical records, laboratory data). So, although retrospective here means that we are using data collected in the past, the direction of the events of interest is forward. This is why they are named "cohort" studies, to evoke a vision of Caesar's army advancing on their enemy. Many studies based on administrative data, such as billing codes or pharmacy records, are of this design.

Some of the well-known examples of prospective cohort studies are The Framingham Study and The Nurses' Health Study, to name two. These are bulky and enormously expensive undertakings, going on over decades, addressing myriad hypotheses. But the returns can be pretty impressive: Just look at how much we have learned about coronary disease, its risk factors and modifiers, from the Framingham cohort. And likewise, the Nurses' Health Study has been running for nearly four decades and has given us reams of information on women's health issues.

This type of a design is known as the "inception cohort," wherein healthy women were enrolled; interviewed about their lifestyle, habits, and health; examined at given intervals; and monitored for the onset of many different diseases. A study like this casts a broad net and then moves forward in time to ask questions about behaviors and other exposures and disease incidence and outcomes. Despite being one of the most fruitful studies of its kind, it is, however, most recognized for its contribution to the confusion over menopausal HRT and, therefore, serves as a vivid illustration of the potential pitfalls of these designs to answer questions related to drug treatment. Based on observational data, for years we prescribed menopausal hormone replacement to prevent such dire consequences of the loss of estrogen as coronary disease. It took only one very well designed and executed extraordinarily large RCT, the WHI-HRT, to turn this impression on its head and for HRT to start fading into the annals of medical history, joining the ranks of therapeutic blood letting as a cure-all. (If you are calling me out on this, you are right: A prior RCT called HERS failed to show any benefit of HRT on recurrent heart attacks.[28] Furthermore, there are still some debates about the WHI-HRT results. You can find some discussion of this in Chapter 8, where we talked about cognitive biases). Case-control and cohort studies are better left for answering questions about such risks as occupational, behavioral, and environmental exposures, which may be ethically difficult or impossible to study

---

[28]Hulley S, Grady D, Bush T, et al. Randomized trial of estrogen plus progestin for secondary prevention of coronary heart disease in postmenopausal women. Heart and Estrogen/progestin Replacement Study (HERS) Research Group. *JAMA* 1998; 280(7):605–613.

in an experimental way. Caution is to be exercised when testing hypotheses about the outcomes of treatment; these hypotheses are best generated in observational studies but tested in interventional ones when feasible.

The one exception to this rule is *pharmacoepidemiologic* studies, which serve as the cornerstone of *pharmacovigilance*, the science of observation for adverse drug events. This exception makes sense if we accept that it is imperative to set a lower bar for detecting harm than benefit. If this seems obscure, it is a bit. In Chapter 20 we try to sidle up to what statistically sets apart desirable and undesirable outcomes, and we delve into some of the philosophical and statistical issues that surround them. The material there will help you grasp the justification for using observational studies to detect adverse signals, particularly when long-term large RCTs are not pragmatic.

There is a feature of the case-control design that I must contrast with a cohort study in order to inform our future discussion of measures of association. In a *cohort study* we begin with a pool of subjects who are all at risk for developing the outcome of interest. For example, if we were interested to learn whether HRT causes breast cancer, we would enroll a certain number of women (let's say 1,000) who do not have breast cancer. Some of these women will be on HRT, while others will not. We would then follow these women over a particular period of time, say 10 years, until some of them develop breast cancer (say 100). Since all of the women belong to the sample group that we selected to represent all similar subjects, the incidence of breast cancer over 10 years in this group, 100 cases per 1,000 women, gives us an idea of the risk of developing this cancer in the population: 10% over 10 years. We can further comment on this risk in the group that took HRT and compare it to the group that did not.

In contrast, a *case-control study* identifies a group of women who are known to have breast cancer (let's say 100). It then goes on to identify a certain number (let's say 100) of controls from among women who are similar in other ways but who do not have breast cancer. It then goes on to compare the prevalence of the exposure in each group, which can lead us to an inference about whether HRT and breast cancer are in any way related. What I hope has become very clear is that because the number of both cases and controls is chosen by the investigators, the total pool of women in the study does not represent all women in a population who are at risk for breast cancer. For this reason, and in sharp contrast to a cohort study and even a cross-sectional study, a case-control design cannot tell us what the frequency of the disease or the exposure in the underlying population is. Therefore, our statistical approach is to utilize the idea of "odds" rather than "risk." This will become important when we talk about measures of association and hypothesis testing.

CHAPTER 16

Interventional Studies

A nd now, on to *interventional* designs, the most
commonly encountered of which is a randomized
controlled trial (RCT). The central feature of a RCT is
that patients are randomly assigned to two or more
groups, each receiving a different intervention, be it a
drug or a device or a package of care. In the context of
the PECOT model, E, the primary intervention under
study, is compared to C, the comparator (see Chapter
13). The difference between this and the observational
design is that the intervention does not happen as a
part of the normal therapeutic encounter but is itself
the experimental exposure.

Because it is thought to be the most accurate way to
establish causality, the RCT has garnered a dispropor-
tionate share of attention. To be sure, matters of effi-

cacy ("Does a particular intervention work statistically better than the placebo under very specific circumstances?") are best addressed with a RCT. One of the distinct shortcomings of this design, however, is its narrow focus on very controlled events, frequently accompanied by examining surrogate outcomes (those that matter more in the laboratory, e.g., blood pressure control) rather than meaningful clinical outcomes (those that matter in real life, e.g., death from stroke). This feature makes the results dubious when translated to the real world. In fact, it is well appreciated that we are prone to see much less spectacular results in everyday practice than in a RCT.

What happens in the real world is termed "effectiveness" and is ideally also addressed via a RCT. However, pragmatically speaking, effectiveness is less amenable to this design. You may see mention of pragmatic or practical clinical trials of effectiveness. A subset of a RCT, practical clinical trials have the following characteristics: "(1) Select clinically relevant alternative interventions to compare, (2) include a diverse population of study participants, (3) recruit participants from heterogeneous practice settings, and (4) collect data on a broad range of health outcomes."[29] All of these char-

_____

[29]Tunis, S. R., Stryer, D. B., & Clancy, C. M. Practical clinical trials: Increasing the value of clinical research for decision making in clinical and health policy. *JAMA* 2003; 290:1624–1632

acteristics set practical trials apart from traditional efficacy RCTs, with the latter usually using placebo as a
comparator in a narrow population and practice setting, focusing on a single outcome or a small handful of
outcomes. While attractive from the perspective of
policy, the ambitious aims of practical clinical trials
make these studies pragmatic in name only, being ex-
ceedingly large and labor- and resource-intensive.
Therefore, few are ever performed. So, in sum, while a
RCT is the best design for inferring a causal relationship, the narrow focus of regulatory trials and high bar-
riers to running practical trials force us to draw
conclusions about real-life safety and effectiveness from
real-world observational, rather than randomized interventional, data.

Our beacon study on this tour of medical literature,
the WHI-HRT, is a great illustration of a practical clinical trial. WHI-HRT is an extraordinarily large RCT in
a broad group of subjects asking a relevant question:
Does menopausal combination (both estrogen and
progesterone) HRT reduce the risk of coronary disease? Several other important outcomes are examined
in the context of HRT exposure. From this perspective,
it met all of the criteria for a practical trial. Up until the
results of this study came out, the evidence from the lab
and from the observational data had demonstrated that
HRT was indeed protective against heart disease, and
millions of women were being prescribed this treatment. It took nearly a decade and over 16,000 women,

one-half treated with HRT and one-half with a placebo, for us to learn that HRT was in fact associated with a substantial **increase** in cardiovascular disease, in addition to breast cancer, strokes, and blood clots. Why such discrepant findings between the observational and interventional data? Well, the answers lie in threats to validity, which we will address in great detail in Chapter 17. This certainly is an illustration of how science works: Sometimes our notions are simply wrong, and they need to be thrown under the bus.

Just a few words about *interrupted time series* studies, as this is the design pervasive in quality improvement literature. You may see these called by various names—interrupted time series, before-and-after, controlled before-and-after, as examples—and each of these carries subtle nuances of its own. A lot of the time, however, these types of studies are commonly referred to as simply before-and-after. The idea is to measure outcomes of interest in a group of patients sampled from a similar population before and after implementation of an intervention, and this is why it is a particularly attractive design for evaluating quality improvement interventions.

Several years ago, the Agency for Healthcare Research and Quality funded a large statewide study in Michigan called the "Keystone Project." Its goal was to test strategies that would help reduce the scourge of healthcare-associated infections. At the helm of this initiative was Peter Pronovost, a young and energetic academic intensivist from Johns Hopkins. After much deliberation and discussion, this herculean organizational effort paid off with stellar data published in the *New England Journal of Medicine*, putting both the resulting checklists and Dr. Pronovost on the healthcare quality map. This most well publicized portion of the project was aimed at eradication of central line–associated blood stream infections (CLABSI).[30] The exposure was a comprehensive evidence-based intervention bundle geared ultimately at building a "culture of safety" in the ICU. The authors call this a cohort design, but the deliberate nature of the intervention arguably puts it into an interventional trial category. Regardless of what we call it, the "before" refers to measurement of CLABSI rates prior to the intervention, while the "after," of course, is following it. There are many issues with this type of design, ranging from confounding to bias, both of which will be addressed in a subsequent chapter. Note that the Keystone study, similar to other studies of its ilk, was not blinded. Why does it matter? Because of a threat we call the "Hawthorne effect": Described initially in the 1950s, this phenomenon essentially refers to the proclivity of humans to improve their performance while being merely observed, regardless of the intervention. We can

---

[30]Pronovost, P. J., Needham, D., Berenholtz, S., et al. An intervention to decrease catheter related bloodstream infections in the ICU. *New England Journal of Medicine* 2006; 355:2725–2732

argue whether or not it matters: After all, so long as there is improvement in quality, is the cause not just of academic interest? I am personally of the opinion that deliberate, expensive, and labor-intensive interventions should only be advocated if we are convinced that they are causing the changes. Others hold to other opinions. But regardless of yours, you need to be aware that you will encounter this design a lot if you read quality and safety literature.

I will not say much about the crossover design, as it is fairly self-explanatory and is relatively infrequently used. Suffice it to say that subjects can serve as their own controls in that they get to experience both the experimental treatment and the comparator in tandem. This is also fraught with many methodological issues, which we will be touching upon in subsequent chapters.

There are other types of study designs that deserve their own categories. Cost-effectiveness studies, decision analyses, and Markov models are some of them, though they lie beyond the scope of the current volume.

CHAPTER 17

Threats to Validity: Bias, Misclassification, and Generalizability

You have heard this many times: No study is perfect. But what does this mean? In order to be explicit about why a certain study is not perfect, we need to be able to name its flaws. And let's face it: Some studies are so flawed that there is no reason to bother with them, either as a reviewer or as an end user of the information. But again, we need to identify these nails before we can hammer them into the study's coffin.

It is the authors' responsibility to include a Limitations paragraph somewhere in the Discussion section, in which they lay out all of the threats to validity and offer educated guesses as to the importance of these threats and how they may be impacting the findings.

Our example of WHI-HRT has an entire subsection with the title "Limitations" in bold letters; such prominence is unusual, but you should find one, albeit without its own label, in every paper somewhere within three to four paragraphs or so of the end of the Discussion. I personally, on principle, will not accept a paper that does not present a coherent Limitations paragraph. However, reviewers are not always this categorical about it, and that is when the reader is on her own. Let us be clear: Even if the Limitations paragraph is included, the authors do not always do a complete job (and this probably includes me, as I do not always think of all the possible limitations of my work); and the reviewers, though helpful, may miss a few as well. So, as in everything, *caveat emptor*!

There are four major threats to validity that fit into two broad categories. They are:

I. Internal Validity
    1. Bias
    2. Confounding/interaction
    3. Mismeasurement or misclassification
II. External Validity
    4. Generalizability

Internal validity refers to whether the study really shows that a certain exposure causes the outcome. This is why RCTs have the highest degree of internal validity, especially when the C is a placebo. The thinking here is that, all other things being equal, the measured effect difference between the treatment under study and the placebo has to be due to the effect of the treatment. For example, in the recent controversy over the effects of antidepressant medications among people with mild depression, this causality has come into serious doubt; that is, it appears much more likely that in this population of patients it is not at all the medication that is causing their symptoms to improve, but rather, a placebo effect. Bias, confounding, and misclassifcation can each cause such a breakdown in the internal validity.

Bias is defined as "any systematic error in the design, conduct, or analysis of a study that results in a mistaken estimate of an exposure's effect on the risk of disease."[31] I think of bias as something that artificially makes the exposure and the outcome occur either together or apart more frequently than they do in reality. For example, the INTERPHONE study, which examined the potential health consequences of cellular phone use, has been criticized for its biased design, in that it defined exposure as at least one cellular phone call every week.[32] Enrolling such light users has two related consequences: (1) They are not representative of

---

[31]Schlesselman, J. J. (2004). Cited in L. Gordis, *Epidemiology*, 3rd ed. (p. 238). Philadelphia, PA: Saunders.

[32]The Interphone Study Group. Brain tumour risk in relation to mobile telephone use: Results of the INTERPHONE international case–control study. *International Journal of Epidemiology* 2010; 39:675–694.

the exposure that is trying to be studied, and (2) the exposure may be so small as to be inconsequential, and therefore no health effects can be detected. This is an example of a selection bias, by far the most common form that bias takes. Another example of a frequent bias is encountered in retrospective case-control studies in which people are asked to recall distant exposures. Take for example middle-aged women with breast cancer who are asked to recall their diets when they were in college. Now, ask a similar group of women without breast cancer. What you are likely to get is the effect, absent in women without cancer, of seeking an explanation for the cancer that expresses itself in a bias in what women with cancer recall eating in their youth. So, a bias in the design can make the association seem either stronger or weaker than it is in reality.

I want to skip over confounding and interaction at the moment, as these threats deserve a chapter of their own. Suffice it to say here that a *confounder* is a factor related to both the exposure and the outcome. An *interaction* is also referred to as effect modification or effect heterogeneity, which means that there may be population characteristics that alter the response to the exposure of interest.

For now, let us move on to *measurement error* and *misclassification*. Measurement error, resulting in misclassification, can happen at any step of the way: it can be in the primary exposure (the one we are most interested in exploring), a confounder, or the outcome of interest. I run into this problem all the time in my research. Since I rely on administrative data for a lot of my studies, I am virtually certain that the codes used for billing routinely misclassify some of the exposures and confounders with which I deal. Take *Clostridium difficile*, the most frequent cause of antibiotic-associated diarrhea, as an example. There is an ICD-9 (billing) code to identify it in administrative databases. However, we know from multiple studies that it is not perfectly sensitive (able to identify disease when disease is present) or perfectly specific (able to identify patients without the disease as not having that disease); it is merely good enough, particularly for making observations over time.

While the ICD-9 example is obvious, other more subtle opportunities for misclassification also exist. This may seem counterintuitive; but even for laboratory values and other diagnostic testing results, there is a certain potential for measurement error, though we, and this includes clinicians, seem to think that these are sacred and immune to mistakes. Indeed, the possibility of error and misclassification is ubiquitous. What needs to be determined by the investigator and the reader alike is the probability of that error. If the probability is high, one needs to understand whether it is a systematic error (for example, a coder is always more likely than not to include *C. difficile* as a diagnosis) or a random error (a coder is just as likely as not to include a *C. difficile* diagnosis). And while a systematic error may result in either a stronger or a weaker association between the exposure and the outcome, a random, or non-differential, misclassification will virtually always reduce the strength of this association.

External validity, synonymous with generalizability, gives us an idea about how broadly the results are applicable. As a concept it helps the reader understand the population to which the results may be applicable. In other words, will the data be applied strictly to the population represented in the study? If so, is it because there are biological reasons to think that the results would be different in a different population? And if that is so, is it simply the strength of the association that can be expected to be different, or is it possible that even the direction could change? In other words, could something found to be beneficial in one population be either less beneficial or even harmful in another? The last question is the reason that we perseverate on this idea of generalizability. Typically, a regulatory RCT, or one designed for the drug approval process, is much less likely to give us adequate generalizability than is, say, a well-designed cohort study. As an example, you may have heard that many studies of cardiovascular diseases have traditionally enrolled predominantly middle-aged men. As a consequence, we know a lot about presentation and treatment of coronary disease in this group and are only now beginning to appreciate its differences among women.

CHAPTER 18

Statistical Analyses: Measures of Central Tendency

You may wonder why I am skipping over *confounding* and *interaction* (they will be treated in Chapter 21) and diving right into the *statistical analyses*. There is a good reason for this: We need to build the ark of some of the more descriptive aspects of data before we plunge into the analytical ocean. So, let's talk about measures of central tendency first.

I have a motto: If you have good results, you do not need fancy statistics. This goes along with the idea in math and science that truth and computational beauty go hand in hand. So, if you see something very fancy that you have never heard of, be on guard for less than spectacular results. This, of course, is just a rule of thumb and, as such, will have exceptions.

The general questions I ask about statistics are:

1. Are the analyses appropriate to the study question(s)?
2. Are these appropriate analyses done correctly?

And here is the systematic way in which I tend to go about answering these questions.

The first thing to establish is the integrity and completeness of the data. If the authors enrolled 365 subjects but were only able to analyze 200 of them, this is suspicious. You should be able to discern how complete the data set was and how many analyzable cases there were. A simple litmus test is that if more than 15% of the enrolled cases did not have complete data for analysis or dropped out for other reasons, the study becomes suspect for a selection bias: The greater the proportion of dropouts, the greater the suspicion, with all the dangerous implications for the internal validity of the results.

Once you have established that the set is fairly complete, move on to the actual analyses. Here, first thing is first: The authors need to describe their study group(s); hence, descriptive statistics. Usually this includes so-called "baseline characteristics," which consist of demographics (age, gender, race), other diseases that are likely to affect the relationship between the primary exposure and the outcome (in the WHI-HRT, they were history of high blood pressure and diabetes, for example), and some measure of the primary condition in question (history of angina or myocardial infarction in the WHI-HRT). Other relevant characteristics may be reported as well, and this is dependent on the study question. As you can imagine, *categorical variables* (variables that have categories, like race, gender, or death) are expressed as proportions or percentages, and *continuous variables* (those that are a continuum, like age) are represented by their measures of central tendency.

It is important to understand *continuous variables* well. There are three major measures of central tendency: mean, median, and mode. Adding all individual values of a particular variable and dividing by the number of values derives the *mean*. So, in a group of 10 subjects, adding all 10 individual ages and then dividing by 10 would yield the mean age. The *median* is the value that occurs in the middle of a distribution. So, if there are 25 subjects with ages ranging from 5 to 65, the median value is the one that occurs in subject number 13 when subjects are arranged in ascending or descending order by age. The *mode*, a measure used least frequently in clinical studies, signifies, somewhat paradoxically, the value in a distribution that occurs most frequently.

Let's focus on the mean and the median. The mean is a good representation of the central value in a normal distribution. This distribution is also referred to as the *bell curve* (yes, because of its shape) or a Gaussian distribution (named after the famous mathematician Karl F. Gauss). In this type of distribution there are roughly equal numbers of points to the left and to the right of the mean value (Figure 2).

For a distribution like the one in Figure 2, it hardly matters which central value is reported, the mean or the median, as they are the same or very similar to one another. Alas, many descriptors of human physiology are not normally distributed but are more likely to be *skewed*, meaning that there is a tail at one end or the other of the curve (Figures 3a and 3b).

In my world of health services research, for example, many values for such variables as length of hospital stay and costs spread out to the right of the center, similar to the graph in Figure 3a. In this type of distribution the

Figure 2 Normal, or Gaussian, distribution. Also referred to as the "bell curve."

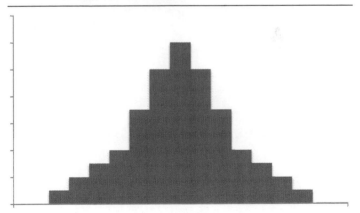

Figure 3a Right-skewed Distribution

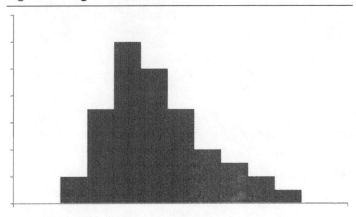

Figure 3b Left-skewed Distribution

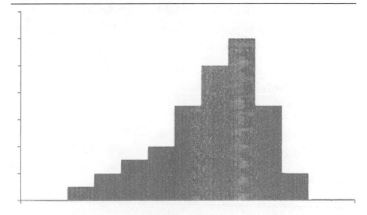

mean and the median values are not the same, and they tell you different things. While the mean gives you an idea of the central tendency of the entire distribution, the median will tell you the central tendency of the majority of the distribution that is tightly clustered at the end opposite the tail. For a distribution similar to the one in Figure 3a (skewed to the right), the mean exceeds the median, whereas for the one in Figure 3b (skewed to the left) the median exceeds the mean. Generally when the results are not distributed normally, the preferred central tendency to report is the median, though for various reasons it is even better when both the mean and the median are reported.

To round out the discussion of central values, we need to say a few words about *scatter* around these values. Because they represent a population and not a single individual, measures of central tendency will have some variation around them that is specific to the population. Variation around the median is usually expressed as the range of the values falling into the central one-half of all the values in the distribution, discarding the 25% at each end, or the *interquartile range* (IQR 25, 75) around the median. For a mean value, this variation is usually represented by the *standard deviation* (SD), though sometimes you will see a 95% *confidence interval,* or 95% CI, as the measure of the scatter. These values represent the stability or precision of our estimates and are important to look for in studies.

It is worth digressing to learn more about what the 95% CI is. If you look at Table 2 in the WHI-HRT paper, at the intersection of the second row and the column called "hazard ratio," you see a number 1.29.

What does this mean? Well, the hazard ratio (discussed in the next chapter) of 1.29 indicates that in this study there was a 29% relative increase in the risk of developing coronary heart disease in the HRT group above the risk seen in the placebo group. But remember, any study represents but a sample of the entire population that it is trying to describe. If the same study was repeated with a different subset of 16,000 women, chances are the observed hazard ratio would have been different. How different? This is the question that the 95% CI is meant to answer. In the column following the heading "Hazard Ratio" in the same row called "Nominal 95% CI," there is a range of 1.02 to 1.63. This 95% interval means that, if we repeated the same experiment 100 times, each time with a different complement of subjects who still represent the population of interest, 95 out of those 100 trials would yield the hazard ratio between 1.02 and 1.63.

CHAPTER 19

Hypothesis Testing and Measures of Association

The scientific method that we generally practice demands that we state a hypothesis prior to conducting a study that will test this hypothesis. The hypothesis is generally advanced as the so-called "null hypothesis" (or H_0), wherein we express our skepticism that there is a difference between groups or that an association between the exposure and the outcome exists. (If you think about it, what I refer to as a "difference" is really the same as the "association" between a given exposure and an outcome. The difference refers to what we observe when comparing the outcome in the group that had the exposure to the one that did not. If there is a difference, then we can say that the exposure is indeed associated with the outcome). So, reflecting back to the specific nutritional question we posed in Chapter 13, the H_0 would be: Consuming 3 cans of sugar-sweetened soda per day does not result in 10% body weight gain over 30 weeks. By starting out with this negative formulation, we set the stage for "disproving" the null hypothesis, or demonstrating that the data support the "alternative hypothesis" (H_A, or the presence of said association or difference). This is where all the measures of association come in, and we will discuss them in greater detail now.

Associations have two important properties: (1) strength, or effect size, and (2) precision. The strength of the association between an exposure and an outcome is most frequently expressed as a relative risk (RR) or an odds ratio (OR): The higher this number, the stronger the association, or the greater the effect size. The RR quantifies the ratio of the outcome among those with the exposure relative to those without (Table 5). In contrast, the OR is the ratio of the odds of disease among those

TABLE 5 Relative Risk Ratio and Odds Ratio Calculation

	Disease present	Disease absent	Total
Exposed	A	B	A + B
Unexposed	C	D	C + D
Total	A + C	B + D	

RR = (A/[A + B]) / (C/[C + D])
OR = (A/B) / (C/D)

with the exposure to the odds of disease among those without. It is also important to understand that the OR, but not the RR, can be calculated in a case-control study, whereas both the RR and the OR can be derived in a cohort study or a RCT. The reason for this, as we discussed in our description of the case-control design in Chapter 15, is that "risk" compares the exposed to the unexposed as a part of the total pool of subjects at risk, while "odds" merely pits those exposed against the unexposed.

To clarify risk versus odds, let's talk about horses: When we hear that Horse A's odds are 1:9 to win, it means that it is expected to lose 9 out of 10 races. This translates to the risk of a loss of 90%. Now, suppose Horse B's odds are 4:6 to win, meaning that, because it is expected to win 4 out of 10 races, and conversely to lose 6 of these 10 races, its risk of a loss is 60%. Now we need to pose a slightly more complicated question: What is the relative risk for Horse B to lose compared to Horse A? In other words, how much more likely than Horse B is Horse A to race to a defeat? Let me introduce you to an invaluable tool that all epidemiologists love, a 2×2 square. Here, the 2×2 square represents the results of ten races for each horse (Table 6).

To calculate the reduction in the odds of a loss for Horse B relative to a loss for Horse A, or the odds ratio, we do the following calculation: $(6 \div 4)/(9 \div 1) = 1.5/9 = 1/6 = 0.167$, or 16.7%. So, the relative reduction in the odds of losing with Horse B compared to Horse A is 100% − 16.7% = 83.3%.

TABLE 6 Odds versus Risk

	Loss	Victory	Total
Horse A	9	1	10
Horse B	6	4	10

And what about relative risk? To calculate the *relative risk*, we would need first to compute the risk of a loss for each horse: For Horse A it is 9 ÷ 10 = 0.9, or 90%; for Horse B it is 6 ÷ 10 = 0.6, or 60%. The relative risk is simply the ratio of these two risks, or (6 ÷ 10)/(9 ÷ 10) = 0.6/0.9 = 0.667, or 66.7%. To calculate the relative risk reduction of a loss for Horse B relative to Horse A, we subtract this value, 66.7%, from 100%, deriving the relative risk reduction of 33.3%.

Now, what do you see when you compare the relative reduction in the odds (83.3%) to the relative reduction in the risk (33.3%) of a loss? A dramatic difference, right? Now, just substitute "treatment A" and "treatment B" for the horses, and substitute "death" for loss of a race. So what are the implications for clinical studies? Is the odds ratio always useless? If it is, why is it used?

Well, the OR is certainly not useless. And mind you, it is the only measure of association available to us in a case-control study. But given our observation in the horse race example, it is important to understand when the OR is a good approximation of the RR; and this is the case when the outcome under study is rare, on the order of 10% or under. When this criterion is not met, the OR will generally overestimate the strength of the association compared to the RR, as we saw in the horse race example. In Table 5, I gave you a general example of a 2×2 table and the formulas that you can use to do your own OR and RR calculations.

The 95% confidence interval (CI) represents the precision of the estimated relationship between the exposure and the outcome. In contrast to the measures of strength, the precision of the estimate goes up as the 95% CI shrinks. The CI can be obtained based on a known distribution that approximates the population in the study (e.g., z distribution, t distribution). It is interpreted in the following way: If the study is repeated 100 times, we have a 95% chance of obtaining a value that is between the bounds of the 95% CI. It is not correct to say "The value we obtained in the study has a 95% chance of being in the interval"—it already either is or is not in that interval. The 95% CI is related to the p value, which we will be discussing later, since both are based on the same distribution.

CHAPTER 20

Statistical Significance, Type I and Type II Errors

This is a great place to discuss the p value, a measure of statistical significance, which will feed our discussion of Type I and Type II errors. First, let us remind ourselves of this simple fact: All studies that we do, no matter how big or small, enroll a finite group of people who presumably represent a larger universe of people with the same characteristic(s) of interest. For example, suppose you wanted to test the hypothesis that, as a general rule, people with brown hair are more likely than people with blond hair to have brown eyes. For obvious reasons you could not possibly enroll the entire universe of people with brown hair and people with blond hair. Therefore, you have to settle for enrolling a "sample" of such people, who will serve as representatives of these populations. This is important, since it illustrates that studies simply try to approximate reality.

Keeping this in mind, let us define the *p* value. The *p* value is a way of checking whether it is more likely that you got your result by chance than by the actual existence of the association. The *p* value is the *probability* that the intergroup difference or association found (in the study), or one that is greater than that, would have been found if in reality there were no difference between the groups. So, a small *p* value is desirable. Failure to disprove the null hypothesis may be because there truly is no difference between the groups being compared (that is, the null hypothesis represents reality) or because we did not find the difference that in fact exists. The latter is essentially a *false negative* result, referred to as the *Type II error*, and can happen for several reasons. The most common of these reasons is a sample size that is too small to detect a statistically significant difference.

I (and others) would argue that the *p* value is the most misunderstood and most misused statistical concept. I am often exasperated by remarks from colleagues who assert that a study was negative by citing the *p* value as proof, in isolation from all other data. It is astonishing how easily highly educated professionals can be so fooled by this sleight of hand. What they do not recall is the true meaning of the *p* value and its checkered history. This value has been in circulation for nearly a century, first described by R. A. Fisher, the father of frequentist statistics. Briefly, *frequentist statistics* assumes equal probabilities for all events, regardless of the potential underlying predisposition to some and not to others. Frequentist statistics are complemented by Bayesian statistics, where the prior probability of an event is key to interpreting any calculation. Nowhere is this distinction more palpable than in the field of preclinical disease identification, which relies on screening large populations of people at low risk for the disease. Thus, for example, because women under 50 years of age have a relatively small chance of harboring breast cancer and because mammography is not a perfectly accurate test, a positive result on a screening mammography is much more likely to represent a false positive than actual disease. Therefore, in clinical situations, it is critical to apply Bayesian rather than frequentist thinking when interpreting data. The p value represents the extreme of frequentist thinking and, thus, misleads more than it informs.

Here are some pitfalls of the p value to avoid. In clinical research we set a high bar for avoiding a *false positive*, or *Type I error*, and a much lower bar for a false negative, a Type II error. The p value is the probability of chance giving rise to the result of the effect size observed or an effect size of a greater magnitude under the circumstances of no real association or difference. For historical reasons we usually set the probability threshold for statistical significance, also referred to as α, at 0.05, meaning that there is a less than 5% likelihood of obtaining the given result or one of greater magnitude by chance if in reality there is no association. This clearly stacks the deck against calling an association positive. In contrast, we are much more willing to obtain a false negative, since many studies set the minimum power to detect the difference where a true difference exists at only 80%. So, in other words, we want to be 95% sure that a positive result is not a false positive association, yet leave ourselves open 20% of the time to miss a true association where one may exist. You see the difference? We are clearly keener to discard associations that do not really exist than to identify those that do. To an untrained eye the difference may be subtle, but it creates a world of philosophical difference in how we approach data.

There are some instances where being overly sensitive to the difference may be beneficial. One of these instances occurs when trying to detect harm rather than benefit. For example, given how ubiquitous some exposures are (e.g., bisphenol A) and how little we know about their long-term health effects (e.g., coronary heart disease), is it fair to discard any association of harm that does not meet the 95% certainty threshold? The same idea applies to the detection of drug-related adverse events, or pharmacovigilance, which we touched on earlier. In this case, despite all the methodological pitfalls that we have outlined so far, lower thresholds for positivity in designs that are less than optimal (e.g., observational studies) help to identify potential signals. In this case caution is definitely the better part of valor, despite an increase in the uncertainties that these methodological considerations create.

I cannot talk about the p value without taking the opportunity to touch on the distinction between "absence of evidence" and "evidence of absence." The difference, though ostensibly semantic, is quite important.[33] While "evidence of absence" implies that studies to look for exposure/outcome associations have been done and done well, have been published, and have consistently shown the lack of such a relationship, "absence of evidence" means that studies examining such associations simply do not exist. Absence of evidence does not absolve the exposure from causing the outcome, yet so often it is confused with the definitive evidence of absence of an effect.

One of the most common reasons for finding no association where in reality one exists, or a Type II error, is, as I have already mentioned, a sample size that is too small to detect a difference. For this reason, in a published study that fails to show a difference between groups, it is critical to ensure that the investigators performed a power calculation. This maneuver, usually found in the Methods section of the paper, lets us know that the sample size is adequate to detect a difference if one exists, thus minimizing the probability of Type II

[33]Altman, D. G. & Bland, J. M. Absence of evidence is not evidence of absence. *British Medical Journal* 1995; 311–485.

error. The trouble is that, as we know, there is a phenomenon called "publication bias." This refers to the scientific journals' reluctance to publish negative results. And while it may be appropriate to reject studies prone to Type II error due to poor design, true negative results must be made public. Until this is done, we will never have the full picture of health and disease. Suffice it to say that the power calculation is of utmost importance, particularly in the face of a negative result.

I will now ask you to indulge me in one more digression. I am sure that in addition to "statistical significance," you have heard of "clinical significance." This is an important distinction, since even a finding that is statistically significant may have no clinical significance whatsoever. Take, for example, a therapy that cuts the risk of a non-fatal heart attack by 0.05% in a certain population. This means that in a population at a 10% risk for a heart attack over 10 years, the intervention will bring this risk on average to 9.95%. (Note that this is *absolute* risk, in contrast to the *relative* risk discussed in the previous chapter.) And though we can argue whether or not this is an important difference to an individual, at the population level, this does not seem all that clinically significant. So, if I have a vested interest and the resources to run a massive trial that will render this minute difference statistically significant, I can do that and then say without blushing that my treatment works. Yet, statistical significance always needs to be examined in the clinical context. This is why it is not enough to read the headlines that tout new treatments.

Along these lines I want to mention one very handy measure, the *number needed to treat* (NNT). The NNT tells you how many people need to be treated in order to get one win. In the preceding discussion of significance, the win is avoiding a heart attack; but it can just as easily refer to avoiding death and other undesirable health events. The NNT calculation is quite simple, but it requires data that are not always easily accessible in a paper, though they should be. The NNT is simply the inverse of the absolute risk difference between the two exposures being compared. So when a drug reduces the rate of heart attacks from 10% to 9.95%, the absolute risk difference is 0.05%, whose inverse is $1 \div 0.0005$, or 2,000. This means that you need to treat 2,000 patients with high blood pressure for 10 years and expose them all to the expense and the potential side effects of the drug in order to avoid 1 heart attack. Conversely, if the absolute reduction were to be from 10% to 5%, the NNT would be 20, a much more reasonable probability of success with much less collateral damage.

As a general rule, the lower the NNT, the better the treatment. But this idea does not have to be limited to "T," or "treat." The same calculation applies to NNI (number needed to *invite* for screening) and to NNH (number needed to *harm*), with some minor distinctions. In the case of mammography screening, the NNI would represent the number of women one needs to invite for screening in order to avoid one death. Again, here a lower number is desirable. Similarly, an example of the NNH is the number of people that one needs to treat with a drug or an intervention in order to have one adverse event, like one diabetic with low blood sugar or one death. In contrast to NNT and NNI, the *higher* the NNH, the better.

A corollary to this is that the lack of statistical significance does not equate with the lack of clinical significance. Given what I said earlier about Type II error, if the difference appears significant clinically (e.g., reducing the incidence of fatal heart attacks from 10% to 5%) but does not reach statistical significance, the result should not be discarded as negative but rather examined for the probability of Type II error.

It is important that we bring this discussion back to the 95% confidence interval, or 95% CI. We talked about its definition and interpretation in Chapter 18, but here I want to point out some of its properties as they relate to statistical significance. Based on the distributions of probabilities from which both these values are derived, the CI is related to the p value. Yet by its very nature, the 95% CI conveys much more information about the statistical significance of the result. Let us go back to the WHI-HRT paper, where statistical significance is indeed expressed as the 95% CI. Table 2 in the paper lists the outcomes of interest for each of the study group, one treated with HRT and the other receiving placebo. One of the top rows lists the "CHD" outcome, and the corresponding cell in the last column gives the interval from 0.85 to 1.97. What does this mean? Well, this gives us an idea of the precision of the point estimate of the risk for CHD (the hazard ratio, HR, in this study) of 1.29 shown in one of the preceding columns. In order to interpret it, we must first recognize that the outcome under evaluation is a categorical one (yes/no, in this case). For a categorical outcome, the value of 1.0 represents the so-called "unity." *Unity* is the point where the risk of the outcome in the presence of the exposure is neither higher nor lower than but is precisely the same as the outcome in the absence of the exposure. It follows then that a value below 1.0 refers to a reduction in the risk and a value above 1.0 to an elevation. While the point estimate for the HR of 1.29 means that the risk for CHD is elevated by 29% in those using HRT, the 95% CI says that if the same trial were to be run 100 times, 95 of those times would yield a HR between 0.85 and 1.97. What this means is that not all 95 out of the 100 trials would demonstrate this harmful association; some of them might come out on the side of benefit, with the number below 1.0. In other words, this 95% CI did not reach statistical significance at the 0.05 (or 5%) level. But the range itself is telling: Most of the values lie above 1.0; and this suggests, at least, that this harmful effect is more likely to be true than not, though we cannot establish this definitively. Could this have been due to a Type II error, where a true association was missed because of a small sample size? It is certainly possible, given the small number of events relative to the gargantuan enrollment of 16,000 subjects, though I am not sure we will ever want to run a larger trial to prove it beyond the shadow of a doubt.

Some additional words about the 95% CI when the outcome is a continuous variable: In this case, as you recall, calculating the slope of the relationship between the exposure and the outcome derives the value for the association. This slope is referred to as the "β-coefficient." For example, when examining the effect of age on blood pressure, we might be faced with an increase of 5 mmHg for every 10 years of increase in age. The slope for this relationship is 0.5 (Figure 4).

Figure 4 Hypothetical Linear Relationship between Age and Systolic Blood Pressure

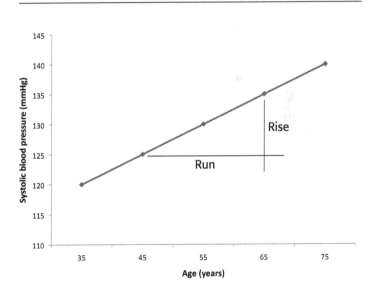

This means that for every year of age there is a 0.5 mmHg rise in the blood pressure. But what if the value for the β-coefficient were a negative number? This would mean that advancing age was actually associated with a reduction in the blood pressure. Similarly, if the 95% CI around this point estimate for the β-coefficient ranged from -0.50 to $+1.50$, this would indicate that this effect did not meet statistical significance at the level of 0.05.

In summary, to be completely clear, when the outcome variable is categorical, in order to reach statistical significance at the level of 0.05, the entire 95% CI needs to be above 1.0 if the risk is elevated or below, when the risk is reduced. Conversely, when the outcome is continuous, statistical significance hinges on the CI's not crossing zero.

There are several rules to be aware of when reading how the investigators tested their hypotheses for statistical significance because different types of variables require different methods. I mention some of these methods here not to give you a complete understanding of when and how they are used, but more for the purpose of building your awareness and recognition of these terms, should you encounter them.

- A categorical variable (one characterized by categories, like gender, race, death, etc.) can be compared using the chi-square test when there is an abundance of events or using the Fisher's exact test when values are scant.

- A normally distributed continuous variable (e.g., age is a continuum that is frequently distributed normally) can be tested using the Student's t-test.
- A variable that has a skewed distribution (e.g., length of hospital stay, costs), requires testing with other methods. Among others, some of the common tests you will encounter are the Mann-Whitney U-test (also called the Wilcoxon rank-sum test), the Kolmogorov-Smirnov test, and the Kruskall-Wallis test.

In short, you do not need to remember any more than this: The test for the hypothesis depends on the variable's distribution. Recognizing some of the situations and test names may be helpful to you in evaluating the validity of a study.

One final frequent computation that you may encounter is *survival analysis*. This is often depicted as a Kaplan-Meier curve and does not have to be limited to examining survival. It is a time-to-event analysis, regardless of what the event is. In studies of cancer therapies we frequently talk about median disease-free survival between groups, and this can be depicted by a Kaplan-Meier analysis. To test the difference between times to event, we employ the log-rank test.

CHAPTER 21

Threats to Validity: Confounding and Interaction

A *confounder* is a factor related to both the exposure and the outcome. Take for example the relationship between alcohol and head and neck cancer (H&N CA). While we know that heavy alcohol consumption is associated with a heightened risk of head and neck cancer, we also know that people who consume a lot of alcohol are more likely to be smokers than those who don't, and smoking in turn raises the risk of H&N CA. So, in this case smoking confounds the relationship between alcohol consumption and the development of H&N CA.

It is virtually impossible to get rid of all confounding completely in any study design, save perhaps for a well-designed RCT, where randomization presumably assures equal distribution of all characteristics; and even there you need an element of luck. In observational studies our only hope to deal with confounding is through statistical manipulation we call "adjustment," as it is virtually impossible to chase it away any other way. To differentiate adjusted results from non-adjusted, you will see various names used for the latter: unadjusted, crude, and nominal (as in the WHI-HRT), to name a few. Even after adjusting, we may still sigh and admit to the possibility of *residual confounding*, meaning that some factors that we failed to identify may remain at play. Nevertheless, going through the exercise is necessary in order to get closer to the true association of the main exposure and the outcome of interest.

There are multiple ways of dealing with the confounding conundrum. Five techniques are used to adjust it away: (1) matching, (2) stratification, (3) regression modeling, (4) propensity scoring, and (5) instrumental variables. By far the most commonly used method is regression modeling; this is what was used in the WHI-HRT. This is a rather complex computation that requires much forethought (in other words, "Professional driver on a closed circuit; don't try this at home"). The frustrating part is that just because the investigators did the regression does not mean that they did it right. Yet word limits for journal articles often preclude authors from giving enough detail on what they did. At the very least they should tell you what kind of a regression they ran and how they chose the terms that went into it. Regression modeling relies on all kinds of assumptions about the data, and it is my personal belief, though I have no solid evidence to prove it, that these assumptions are not always met.

And here are the specific commonly encountered types of regressions and when each should be used:

1. **Linear regression.** This is a computation used for outcomes that are continuous variables, or ones on a continuum of numbers, like age, for example. This technique's main assumption is that the exposure and the outcome are related to each other in a linear fashion. The resulting beta coefficient is the slope of this relationship if it is graphed, that is, the rate of change of Y relative to X (or rise over run, as any middle schooler would tell you, as shown in Figure 4).

2. **Logistic regression.** This is done when the outcome variable is categorical, or fits into two or more categories, like gender, for example, or death or race. The result of a logistic regression is an adjusted odds ratio (OR). It is interpreted as an increase or a decrease in the odds of the outcome occurring due to the presence of the main exposure. Thus, an OR of 0.66 means that there is a 34% relative reduction in the odds (used interchangeably with risk, though this is not quite accurate) of the outcome due to the

presence of the exposure. Conversely, an OR of 1.34 means the opposite, or a 34% relative increase in the odds of the outcome if the exposure is present. (See Chapter 19 for a fuller discussion of odds ratios.)

3. **Other generalized linear models (GLM).** Although a detailed discussion of GLMs is beyond the scope of this book, I need at least to mention their existence. They serve many different needs, and one of their most important functions is to give a true measure of risk for a categorical variable in a study design other than a case-control. As I already said, much of the time in medical literature you will see odds ratios reported as a measure of risk, yet odds and risk are not identical (I illustrated this in Chapter19). A GLM is a measure of risk, not odds. It may be confusing that despite being called "linear," GLMs can be applied to categorical variables. Yet this is the case, and you need to be aware of it.

4. **Cox proportional hazards.** This is a common type of model developed for a time-to-event, also known as "survival," analysis even when we are not talking about life and death, but, say, length of stay in the hospital. You will recognize that this is the analysis used in the WHI-HRT. The resulting value is a hazard ratio (HR). Here is another example: the relationship between central line–associated blood stream infection

(CLABSI) and length of stay in the hospital. In this example, a HR of, say, 1.8 means that CLABSI confers an 80% increase in the risk of remaining in the hospital longer. To me this tends to be a problematic technique in terms of assumptions, as it requires that the risk of an event stay constant throughout the time frame of the analysis. And how often does this hold true? For this reason the investigators should be explicit about whether or not they tested for the assumption of proportional hazards and, if they did, whether this assumption was met.

Let's now touch briefly upon the other techniques that help us to unravel confounding. *Matching* is obvious: It is a process of matching subjects with the primary exposure to those without exposure in a cohort study, or subjects with the outcome to those without in a case-control study, based on certain characteristics, such as age, gender, comorbidities, and disease severity, to name a few of the most common ones. By its nature, matching reduces the amount of analyzable data and, thus, reduces the statistical power of the study. ("Statistical power," or just "power," as we discussed in Chapter 20 refers to the study size necessary to detect an association between the exposure and the outcome where one exists). So, it is best left to a case-control setting, where it actually improves the efficiency of enrollment.

Stratification is the next technique. The word *stratum* means "layer," and stratification refers to describing what happens to the layers of the population of interest with and without the confounding characteristic. In the earlier example of smoking confounding the alcohol and H&N CA relationship, stratifying the analyses by smoking (comparing the H&N CA rates among drinkers and non-drinkers in the smoking group separately from the non-smoking group) can divorce the impact of the main exposure from that of the confounder on the outcome. An entry for this stratification in a table would look something like what is in Table 7.

This method has some distinct intuitive appeal, though it gets rapidly cumbersome the more strata that need to be examined.

Propensity scoring is gaining popularity as an adjustment method in the medical literature. A propensity score is essentially a number, usually derived from a regression analysis, describing the propensity of each subject for a particular exposure. So, in terms of smok-

TABLE 7 Example of Stratification: Risk for H&N CA Based on Exposure to Alcohol, Stratified by Smoking

		H&N CA
Smokers	Drinkers	A%
	Non-drinkers	B%
Non-smokers	Drinkers	C%
	Non-drinkers	D%

ing, we can create a propensity score based on other common characteristics that predict smoking. We take advantage of the presence of some of these characteristics also in people who are non-smokers to yield a similar propensity score in the absence of this exposure. In turn, the outcome of interest can be adjusted in several ways for the propensity for smoking. One common way is to match smokers to non-smokers based on the same (or similar) propensity scores and then examine their respective outcomes. This allows us to understand the independent impact of smoking on, say, the development of coronary artery disease. As is true for all modeling, the devil is in the details. Some studies have indicated that many papers that employ propensity scoring as the adjustment method do not do this correctly. So, again, questions need to be asked and details of the technique elicited. There is just no shortcut to evaluating statistics.

Finally, a couple of words about instrumental variables. This tool comes to us from econometrics. An *instrumental variable* is one that is related to the exposure but not to the outcome. One of the most famous uses of this method was published by a fellow you may have heard of, Mark McClellan,[34] in which he looked at the proximity to a cardiac intervention center

---

[34]Mark McClellan is a physician and an economist. He is a former commissioner of the Food and Drug Administration and a former chief administrator of the Centers for Medicare and Medicaid Services.

as the instrumental variable in the outcomes of acute coronary events.[35] Essentially, he argued, the randomness of whether or not you are close to a center "randomizes" you to the type of treatment you get. His argument was based on the fact that people who live in close proximity to a medical center with interventional capabilities, such as cardiac catheterization and surgery, are more likely to receive these interventions during a heart attack than those who live close to centers without such capabilities. Incidentally, in this study he showed that invasive interventions were responsible for a very small fraction of the long-term outcomes among people with heart attacks. I have not seen this method used that much in the literature I read or review, but I am intrigued by its potential.

And now, to finish out this topic, let's talk about interaction. *Interaction* is a term mostly used by statisticians to describe what epidemiologists call "effect modification" or "effect heterogeneity." It is just what the name implies: There may be certain secondary exposures that either potentiate or attenuate the impact of the main exposure of interest on the outcome. Take the triad of smoking, asbestos, and lung cancer. We know that the cumulative risk of lung cancer among

[35]McClellan, M., McMeil, B. J., & Newhouse, J. P. Does more intensive treatment of acute myocardial infarction in the elderly reduce mortality? Analysis using instrumental variables. *JAMA* 1994; 272:859–866.

smokers exposed to asbestos is far higher than the sum of those two risks. Thus, asbestos modifies the effect of smoking on lung cancer. So, to analyze those smokers exposed to asbestos together with those who were not exposed will result in an inaccurate measure of the association of smoking with lung cancer: Among smokers it will yield a weaker association and among non-smokers a stronger association than those that exist in reality. More important, failing to test for such an important potential interaction would steer us away from detecting this very important augmenter of tobacco's carcinogenic potential. To deal with this, we need to be aware of the potentially interacting exposures and either examine the effect of the main exposure of interest on the outcome in the presence and the absence of the modifying exposure separately (stratification) or work the interaction term (usually constructed as a product of the two exposures, in our case smoking and asbestos) into the regression modeling. In my experience as a peer reviewer, interactions are rarely explored adequately. In fact, I am not even sure that everyone understands the importance of recognizing this phenomenon. This is one area where improvement is critical.

CHAPTER 22

Study Results and Conclusions

Up until now we have focused on the clarity of the question, study design, and statistical methodologies. Now let's spend a little time thinking about the results and the conclusions of the study. The questions posed in the previous chapters should guide you in your critical appraisal of the study. Although sometimes difficult, the answers to these questions will help you understand how the results of the study should (or should not) impact practice.

There is a series of additional questions that I pose when I review the results and conclusions of any paper. The answers to these questions arise directly or indirectly out of the concepts we have discussed throughout this book. Some of them are drawn from "Primers" available from the American College of Physicians in their *Effective Clinical Practice* series, and most are self-explanatory.[36]

1. **Has the study answered the question it posed?**
   a. Are the results clearly stated?
   b. Do they match the stated study aims?
   c. Are the results interpreted correctly?
   d. What are the results' direction, magnitude (effect size), precision, and generalizability?
   e. Are they examined in the context of the limitations of the study?
   f. Are results under- or overstated?
   g. Is the outcome the result of the exposure?

2. **Is the study reporting appropriate, transparent, and complete?**
   Luckily, there are guidelines that have been published on best practices for reporting studies that are relatively design specific. (Some of them have really interesting acronyms; my personal favorite is MOOSE!) These are readily available on the web for your reading pleasure (see Table 8). One thing that is worth saying: If you don't get what the investigators did, chances are you are not the only one because the authors failed to make their paper clear enough.

---

[36]American College of Physicians. Primers. Effective Clinical Practice. Available at http://www.acponline.org/clinical_information/journals_publications/ecp/primers.htm

TABLE 8 Reporting Guidelines by Type of Study Design

Acronym	Study type	Reference
CONSORT	Randomized trials	http://www.consort-statement.org/
MOOSE	Meta-analyses of observational studies	http://jama.ama-assn.org/content/283/15/2008.full
QUORUM	Meta-analyses of RCTs	http://www.ncbi.nlm.nih.gov/pmc/articles/PMC2674183/
RATS	Qualitative research	http://www.biomedcentral.com/ifora/rats
STARD	Diagnostic test studies	http://www.stard-statement.org/

3. **Are the study conclusions valid? Are they valuable?**

Finally, you have to decide on the validity of what the study claims to have demonstrated and what it actually demonstrated. More important, are the results valuable? If this is a study that shows a clinically insignificant change in the outcome with very strong statistical significance, I would argue that it may be less valuable than one that demonstrates a large and clinically significant impact on the outcome but somewhat misses the statistical significance hurdle (you have to be careful here to base your judgment on the importance of the outcome, the plausibility of the association, the importance of the outcome, and the margin by which the statistical significance was missed).

Any new study needs to be put in the context of the existing body of knowledge. Fortunately, many publications and services, ranging from the Cochrane Collaboration to the *Journal of Evidence-based Medicine* to many professional organizations, such as the American College of Cardiology, the American College of Chest Physicians, and many other guideline-developing organizations, do the job of locating, appraising, and synthesizing the evidence for you. And truly, this is necessary, in view of the sheer volume of information generated daily, weekly, and monthly. And given all the pitfalls along the way, it is clearly important to be an educated consumer of medical information.

CODA

Only the Beginning

We have come to the end of this introduction to critical evaluation of medical literature. I hope that you have found it helpful and accessible. We covered a lot of material, from how to ask an important and answerable question; to how studies should be designed, executed, and reported; to some of the most nagging issues in science and philosophy. This has been a surprisingly far-reaching journey, where we even touched on such controversial esoterica as p values, Bayesian thinking, and uncertainty.

Some seasoned authors have a simple recommendation for budding writers: If you want to be a writer, write. My advice to you now is similarly simple: If you want to get good at reading medical literature critically, read.

Index

33521262R00104

Made in the USA
Lexington, KY
28 June 2014